The Food Tree

www.Amazon.com

2 4 6 8 9 7 5 3 1

First edition

Copyright © 2008 Ranveig Elvebakk, M.D.
All rights reserved.
ISBN: 0-615-14427-6
ISBN-13: 978-0615144276

Visit www.booksurge.com to order additional copies.

RANVEIG ELVEBAKK, M.D.

THE FOOD TREE

HOW TO DUMP THE DIETS, LOSE WEIGHT, AND TAKE BACK YOUR HEALTH PERMANENTLY

EDITED BY ELIZABETH KESSLER

2008

This Book Is For Trond Rune And Annette.
For My Father And Mother, Olai And Johanna Elvebakk, Who
Gave Me The Curiosity To Search And The Strength To Persist.
For My Brother, Roald, Who Was One Of My First Patients To
Change His Life Using The Food Tree.
And For All My Patients Who Changed Theirs—You Are All Part
Of This Book.

TABLE OF CONTENTS

CHAPTER 1
Good Health and Normal Weight are for Everyone!

Whether your weight is optimal or you're overweight and struggling, you need to know this: From now on, you are granted diet amnesty! Dump the food pyramid. Dump dieting. Dump whatever you're doing if it isn't working for you. You can end the struggle and make peace with food and your weight.

This will become clear to you when you understand the basic principles of nutrition laid out for you in the Food Tree.

If you are at your best weight, you'll stay there eating this way. If you need to lose weight, you'll gravitate toward normal weight effortlessly. If you're underweight, you need to know why, since many illnesses start with weight loss. If you're otherwise healthy, the Food Tree can be adjusted to help you move toward optimal weight in a healthy way.

Good Health Is Not Complicated

Our bodies and nutrition operate on known biochemical principles, making eating a scientific issue. It doesn't follow your astrological sign, blood type, or religious bent. It follows laws that can be understood and used. Best of all, they can be explained. This book does exactly that.

We insist on living in the dark ages of diets, which are nothing but myths clouding a scientific subject. Diets are fads that change like fashions, which is why they're doomed to fail. Meanwhile, the biochemistry of our bodies and nutrition hasn't changed much since we evolved. We've had plenty of time to figure it out—and we actually have!

There's no great mystery to giving your body what it needs to function well, though we keep acting as if there is. Medicine neglects and misunderstands nutrition, leaving you to suffer confusion among countless diets and weight-loss gurus. You're also at the mercy of politicians and economic interests who don't want the facts known. This is abysmal, since nutrition is the cornerstone of good health. If we can put a man on the moon, we can explain the laws of nutrition to you and teach you how to eat. You need to know how your body functions, the difference between food and nonfood, and how your brain works with all of this. Then you need the support to do it. We're going to demystify it and lay it out for you. Rather than show you what *not* to do, we're going to show you exactly what to do, why, and how. It's all known.

Obesity Is a Health Problem That Creates Other Health Problems!

Obesity is more than extra fat that weighs you down. It's an inflammatory disease linked to a multitude of illnesses, from arthritis to eczema. When you lose weight, the inflammation in your body is reduced at the cellular level, and associated conditions, known as metabolic illnesses, improve or disappear as a result.

Good nutrition can reverse obesity-related conditions, including diabetes, high blood pressure, high cholesterol, arthritis, asthma, eczema, psoriasis, chronic fatigue, sleep apnea, polycystic ovarian disease, indigestion, fatty liver, and muscle/joint pain. People suffering from migraine headaches or depression may find that their condition improves dramatically or their symptoms disappear. Nutrition can't reverse permanent tissue damage—if you've had a heart attack or a stroke, the damage is there. But eating properly can keep more damage from occurring. To reclaim health can take time—anywhere from weeks to years (in severe cases). But it can be done.

Starting with type 2 diabetes, most cases can be reversed in short order. There is simply no reason to allow metabolic illnesses to make you a chronic patient when you can stop them in their tracks!

My patients normalize their blood sugar and lower their cholesterol and blood pressure enough to get off medication safely in months. Many of the major illnesses, even some forms of cancer, are linked to obesity. Losing weight will lessen your health risks across the board. You'll be glad you did.

Obesity's Huge Price Tag

Obesity has a huge cost in terms of actual dollars. Being obese is expensive. This "fat tax" affects everyone who's overweight. You pay more for insurance, you spend more time at the doctor's office, and you even make less money than your slim counterparts do. When you're obese, the cost isn't merely cosmetic. Your wallet really takes a beating: you make less and spend more. There's considerable evidence that obese workers are paid less than workers of normal weight.

Then there's your food budget. Most of my patients who use the Food Tree end up eating wonderful food at equal or lower cost because they stop spending incessantly on junk food and become full on much less.

Nearly everyone who loses weight says that the world looks different. The control they feel in their lives is projected to the world around them. Many tell me that they have a new expense: social engagements they've long been hiding from. This is priceless quality of life.

The Food Tree: Simple Science Will Reclaim Your Health

The Food Tree draws from a colorful chapter of nutrition history, including the work of mavericks such as Drs. Linn, Atkins, and Stillman, who recognized that good health depends on harnessing your body's insulin production. They saw the damaging effects of refined sugars, and recognized the role of protein in supporting lean body mass and regulating hunger. They understood that proteins and carbohydrates play a dominant role in regulating health, though the finer points of their biochemistry and interrelationship weren't yet known. They didn't understand the crucial role of fat and its intricate interplay with insulin in the overall balance of nutrients that keeps us healthy. We've advanced our understanding greatly and have actually mapped these connections. This allows us to approach nutrition not as the "high something and low the other" diet, but as the *balance* you need to become healthy and stay that way. It also allows us to show all this to you, so you can use it.

That's exactly what the Food Tree does. It gives you the keys to setting your weight thermostat with food, and creating a weight setpoint that you can change with what you eat. You can use the setpoint to gain, lose, or maintain the same weight. It gives you a precise, step-by-step formula—a real prescription for how to do that. How fast you do it depends on how you design and follow your Food Tree, and how active you are. The issue isn't speed, but the power of finding the formula. The rest will follow.

You can't change what's happened to you in the past—the misinformation you were given, the diets you tried, or the weight roller coaster you've been on. But you can change your future. You can eat well and achieve optimal weight. You can rid yourself of a host of illnesses. You can do it all with good, balanced nutrition. Best of all, you can forever dump the notion that you have to be hungry and suffer to lose weight. It's just not true!

If you're struggling to maintain or lose weight, use the Food Tree.

If you're tired of counting calories, use the Food Tree.

If you want to improve or reverse metabolic illnesses, increase your energy, and restore your health, use the Food Tree.

You'll see that the Food Tree is the information you need to reclaim health. As a patient of mine said, "I've dumped my library of diet books along with fifty pounds. I'm eating, I'm never hungry, I feel great—and I will never diet again!"

It's also well recognized that there's another component to weight and health: We know that our thoughts and emotions influence our bodies. Many people's thoughts get in the way of their health. If that's part of your weight problem, we give you information to rethink this relationship. The Food Tree will teach you how to change your thoughts about food. You might not realize it, but your thoughts determine your weight. This is what's known as *integrative medicine.*

The Power of Mind Technologies

The ancients believed that we all have a constant inner dialogue going on between the voices that want change and those that say we can't change for whatever reasons. We really can't ask our bodies to change if we don't believe change is possible. That's why I work with mind technologies as a big part of the Food Tree. When we believe that we're capable of success, we give ourselves permission to achieve it.

You *can* break your helplessness and introduce powerful new ways of looking at your body and food. You can apply these to any area of your life. You might be familiar with the recent wave of "positive thinking" in the media. Perhaps you're already using similar techniques in your life. They've been there all along. I've specifically adapted them to nutrition, and have been using them very successfully for many years to change my patients' relationship with food.

If you're looking to understand the relationship of your body, mind, and food, read on.

Your Body, the Magnificent Machine

Your poor, overweight, ailing body doesn't want to be beaten into submission with another diet. Neither does it want to weigh 300 pounds and be flooded with the latest high-tech, high-priced supplement or wonder-vitamin to no avail. Research shows that mega doses of vitamins are mostly wasted, and in some cases harmful. Your body wants you to recognize what it needs, stop pummeling it with garbage, and start respecting it by giving it food. It wants to be fed and cared for—it wants your understanding and friendship. No hunger, no suffering diet, just normal weight and good health. This is not about depriving you or taking away your food. If you're overweight and eating badly, you're already deprived of food! Next time you treat yourself to a heaping dose of refined sugar, think about this: *This treat is no treat.* You are "treating" your body to metabolic garbage that it cannot process, depriving it of the building blocks it needs to keep you strong and healthy. *This treat is deprivation.* Conversely, when you eat food, you're treating your body to good health. *That is a treat!* Your body isn't deprived of anything except myths about needing sugar. Sorting out food versus garbage is key to understanding nutrition. That allows you to recognize your body through information. With good nutrition your body stops struggling and becomes what you want it to be because you give it what it needs. I've taught thousands of patients to do this. Would you fill your car's fuel tank with sewer water—and then dislike it if it didn't start? Do you know how many patients come to me complaining that they hate their bodies, but give no thought to how their bodies got that way? The amazing thing is that, whatever you do to it, your body starts—over and over again. Your body has an enormous reserve capacity, but it has no voice to ask you for what it needs. It only reacts to what you give it. If you look in the mirror and in your medicine cabinet, you know what you're giving your body to work with.

Finally, we'll look at making weight loss stick—or why it doesn't. Since this is not understood and is rarely discussed, it's about time we did.

To start, meet some members of my family, genetic and otherwise, who'll testify to what can happen when you're on the Food Tree.

One of the first patients to test my theories was my brother Roald. Until some ten years ago he considered himself healthy. Then he called me with shocking news: His doctor had diagnosed him with diabetes and very high cholesterol, along with being thirty-five pounds overweight. The doctor was teaching him "how to live with diabetes." Roald had other plans. He called me wanting to learn "how to live *without* diabetes."

I put him on the Food Tree and he quickly lost most of the excess weight. His diabetes partly reversed, but not completely. He was as disappointed as I was, but he stuck with the Food Tree. As he saw it, he felt so much better that he really didn't want to go back to being a "garbage can." He also understood that if he went back to his previous eating, his diabetes would worsen. His would turn out to be the most stubborn case of diabetes I've dealt with. While most of my patients test normal for blood sugar within months, it took Roald four years to normalize all his blood sugars, but gradually it happened. He just recently visited his doctor, who refused to believe that Roald was ever diabetic!

Roald's cholesterol has persisted, but a small dose of medication keeps it down. My brother clearly has the worst genes in the family, since my cholesterol and blood sugar are normal. Scientifically, though, we know this: As his sister, I, by definition, have abnormal sugar metabolism. If we started eating large quantities of sugar, I might well test as pre-diabetic and he would be diabetic again. Since that's not an option, we both do the Food Tree and live our lives as well people.

Before the Food Tree, vanity, diets and deprivation kept me thin, inadvertently allowing me to avoid any blood-sugar issues. I feel so lucky that I needn't do those things anymore. I can eat, and I don't have to worry about ever having diabetes because my lifestyle prevents it. Genes are not destiny!

Next is Richard, my brother-in-law, living a stressful New York life in law and politics. He was beginning to project the image of too much of "the good life." Some fifty pounds overweight and with high blood pressure, he had consulted several famous gurus and taken more wonder supplements than he could remember, all to no avail. When he came to San Francisco for a visit, he was heavier than ever, bloated, short of breath, exhausted, and on two blood-pressure medications.

At this point he was willing to try anything—even listen to me! I spent two hours introducing him to the Food Tree. He went back to New York and dropped twenty-five pounds in short order. The bloating diminished and his blood pressure dropped to a one-medicine problem. He has kept the weight off and in Switzerland for a friendly amateur skating competition, he clocked his personal best. I'm urging him to take off the remaining twenty-five pounds and discontinue his second blood pressure medication, which I'm sure he will. His testimonial: "Amazing. No one has ever shown me nutrition this way. I feel so much better, and it's easy!"

Some of Our Leading Ladies

Francesca was sixty-nine and bent over in pain when she walked into my office. She was only fifteen pounds overweight, but suffered terrible chronic fatigue. I started her on the Food Tree. Two weeks later she came back declaring, "I haven't felt this great in ten years!"

Two weeks later and six pounds lighter, she was flying high. Three months into the Food Tree, she had lost fifteen pounds. She said, "What chronic fatigue?" For her seventieth birthday she was traveling the world. These days she spends her money on pampering herself rather than on medical bills.

She wanted me to be sure to tell you this: "Your weight and nutrition are things you can control—and when you do, your whole life changes. I only wish I'd learned it sooner. It is most important that young people learn the Food Tree. It would save them a lot of suffering."

Francesca is a poster girl for helping yourself, and one of several patients who have vastly improved or cured their chronic fatigue using the Food Tree.

Susan, a twenty-something dancer, felt she was overweight for her profession. In reality her weight was normal, but she also suffered from migraines and wanted to try an elimination diet for those.

We designed Susan's Food Tree, and within weeks her migraines were all but gone! Her weight didn't change, but her shape did—she exchanged fat for muscle, and slimmed down till she was perfectly happy with her weight. This illustrates the points I make in chapter 3 about the relationship between nutrition and size, and nutrition's effect on neuro-biochemistry. I have helped several patients like Susan, who just need to change their body composition by changing their eating.

A friend confided in me about her lifelong stomach problems and diverse food intolerances. She had seen a host of doctors who'd never found any definite diagnosis. Thin and athletic, she eats "what she wants." That included a lot of junk food. I told her that what she wanted might not be what her body wanted, and put her on an easygoing dairy/gluten-free Food Tree. Within weeks her stomach pains were gone and she felt great. Since she works in the PR industry, I hope she'll help others by giving the Food Tree credit for changing the way she feels.

Speaking of helping others, one day I walked into the neighboring medical offices in my building to introduce myself and what I do. The personnel I met were generally under-whelmed, but the patients who overheard what I said asked for my card! People don't know they can heal themselves with food, and many of them would like that information. The numbers in my office over the years indicate that 10–30% of metabolic patients would make permanent changes in their lives if they were taught to use the Food Tree. That's a lot of lives changed and medical costs saved!

I worked with a medical receptionist who told me she couldn't get pregnant because of polycystic ovarian syndrome. I put her on the Food Tree and told her to be careful what she wished for. In three months she was pregnant.

Endocrinologists now use the sugar-lowering drug Metformin as a fertility drug. It's not a fertility drug—it lowers blood sugar. Enough said? Keep your blood sugar low and lots of good things can happen.

CHAPTER 2
The Toxic Addictive Connection
Refined Sugars and Grains—Toxic Waste for Your Body

Over the past forty years, we've become increasingly obese and unhealthy. We've also become addicted to a man-made toxic substance and have been brainwashed into calling it food.

This toxin is sugar. In biochemical terms, this includes refined sugars and grains. Sugar consists of more or less complex variations of the basic simple glucose molecule, collectively known as carbohydrates. These come in many guises, and you need to know what they are. Recognizing the toxic ones, and treating them as the toxins they really are, is crucial to reclaiming your health.

The difference is that the natural sugars in vegetables, legumes, and some fruits are absorbed slowly and work as foodstuffs. These are called complex carbohydrates. Refined carbohydrates are the sugars that are rapidly absorbed into your body, raising your insulin level, and making your metabolism produce pro-inflammatory substances. The more refined, the more sugar power—and the more inflammation. This is a metabolic process that is fundamental to our health, and you need a working knowledge of it. You eat sugar and it raises insulin, which turns your cells into inflammatory factories—especially fat cells, and especially those that sit around your waist. This is why that "spare tire" is dangerous.

Sugars come in different guises. Grains, cereal, pasta, bread, rice, and, of course, sugar, are all sugars to your body. Yes, I said sugars. So much for the idea of eating grains for complex carbs. Let me explain this once and for all: If you eat 6 oz. of whole barley (and who does?) your Glycemic Index (GI) is now 22. Crack that barley, and what pours out of the shell is a sugar to the body, registering 50 and above on the GI scale (depending on how finely it is milled.) If used as food, this can easily become toxic to your body! If you want to be healthy, you need to recognize sugar regardless of how it's dressed. You'll find a full explanation of the biochemistry of sugars in chapter 4. You'll also find the GI scale of the most common carbs starting on page 118 of the appendices.

We Were Not Meant to Eat Garbage!

Our digestive tracts were laid down some 100,000 years ago. Our ancestors had little refined sugar in their diet—sugar came only from fruit and perhaps a bit of honey now and then. Anthropologists tell us that metabolic illnesses showed up about the time we learned to grow grains, and worsened with the refining of sugar. When we figured out how to turn sugar into massive amounts of liquor we branched out into alcohol problems. We might eat more sugar in a few days than our forebears ate in a lifetime. Sugar consumption statistics are misleading, in that they don't count disguised sugars. For starters, we live on bread products (derived from grains) as a basic food group. Remember: bread is a refined carbohydrate. And we buy 50 million soft drinks of one particular brand every day.

It's no wonder we're experiencing a dramatic increase in diabetes—our bodies simply weren't made to handle the sugar load. Understanding the relationship between sugar/insulin and metabolic illness will make it clear why we suffer ill health when we ignore these facts.

The Toxic Addictive Cousins

People used to talk about "demon rum." You've been warned that you'll suffer if you don't understand that alcohol is toxic. But we aren't recognizing its demon cousin—sugar. Consumed in large quantities, sugar is just as deadly as alcohol. Chemically, sugar is simply unfermented alcohol. Why do we consume so much of it, and why don't we understand its deadly potential? Because instead of being represented as the health threat it really is, it's foisted upon us as a food group, making it the most insidious of all toxins. What makes it even more menacing is its great potential for physical addiction (see the addiction curve in chapter 3.) In that sense, sugar is really a drug—and a toxic one, just like cousin alcohol. And this is why we can't stop eating it! Chapter 3 will fully acquaint you with the addictive potential of sugar through insulin. Chapter 6 will look at the psychological addiction and at the behavioral side of things.

Our parents gave us more sugar than they ate as children, and we're giving our children even more. Meanwhile, the alarming message is shouting at us: the runaway epidemic of metabolic illness.

Public Enemy #1

The blame can be laid at the feet of the sugar and food industry, the pharmaco-medical-industrial complex, and the leaders and politicians who support the status quo. Since refined sugars took over our diets in the early 1960s, we've burgeoned into a society of the overweight and obese.

While doctors have advised their patients to lower their intake of sugar for years, they don't even know what sugar is. Meanwhile, more and more prepared foods come with sugar already added. The food industry has decided that the more sugar they put in food, the more you'll buy—and they're right!

Have you ever tried to tell an alcoholic that alcohol is bad? It's like telling the joking, self-professed sugar addict that this is not cute. Drinking alcohol used to be cute, even elegant, remember? Our ignorance and denial are showing, and it keeps us victimized. We're not really willing to see the situation for what it is, and continue to eat more and more sugar. Candy and soda are every teenager's fast fix. As processed foods have grown ever more laden with sugar, childhood obesity has become more the norm than the exception. Bad news about the epidemic is everywhere you look today.

Our reaction is to restrict soda in school vending machines while we take our cholesterol medication, communicating to our kids that we want them to do something we can't. And we're saying little about what our poor kids should do instead—and what we should do along with them—the Food Tree.

The Sugar Stunner

At Johns Hopkins in September 2005, Selvin, Coresh, Golden, et al., dropped a little-noticed bombshell into the discussion of the causes of heart disease. They showed that blood sugar predicts risk for heart disease better than any other known risk factor in non-diabetics, that is, people with "normal" blood sugar. We should have known. Khaw's UK study in 2001 showed the same thing. It is further confirmation of more than two decades' worth of studies linking blood sugar and metabolic illness.

It makes perfect biochemical sense, and you'll learn why throughout this book.

Because of all the medical research and practice pointing to sugar as the major trigger of metabolic illness, the Food Tree is geared toward getting all dangerous sugar out of your life and keeping your blood sugar as low normal as possible.

Will the Real Stunner Stand Up Please

Medicine keeps grappling with an apparent paradox: Blood sugar is at the center of metabolic illness, yet lowering it by medications does not lower the risk of other metabolic illness or cardiovascular disease. In fact, aggressively treating it may increase the risks.

We actually have the data to understand why: While sugar is directly toxic to blood vessels, it is not sugar that starts the inflammatory chain that leads to metabolic illness, it is insulin. Insulin is one of the, if not the main regulator of the production of pro-inflammatory substances.

We predictably see that if we lower insulin (which by inference means lowering our blood sugar and weight) we also lower cardiac risk, cholesterol, blood pressure and the other manifestations of metabolic syndrome.

This data comes from bariatric surgery, which reverses diabetes in weeks to months because of the rapid weight loss.

Since research suggests this is true at non-diabetic blood sugar levels as well, this speaks of a regulatory mechanism for blood sugar/insulin that is finely tuned, and the lower we keep our insulin, the better we are off.

What is the consequence of all this? It is that type 2 diabetics should know that aggressive treatment with insulin and insulin-promoting medications may be dangerous to their health. As may bariatric surgery be, for reasons cited elsewhere in this book. But nutrition is not. The Food Tree has safely reversed diabetes for ten years by the G-I curve on page 28. Everyone should understand this curve.

Being healthy is the least dangerous thing to your health!

The Food Pyramid—A Slippery Slope

The USDA Food Pyramid of 1992 was a setback in nutrition that has had serious consequences. Unscientific and arbitrary, it put us right on the addiction fast track. We were told to eat 6–11 servings of cereal, bread, rice, potatoes, and pasta as the base of our nutrition—low fat, of course. Instead of fat, the base of this diet is refined sugar, which raises the body's insulin to dangerous levels and causes weight gain and metabolic complications, not to mention sugar-addiction. This is exactly what we're seeing. Our health is spinning out of control, with no end in sight.

The Price Is *Not* Right

We talked about the price of obesity to the obese person, but since most of us are overweight, we're becoming a society of lifestyle patients from an early age. Meanwhile, the pool of well people is shrinking and we're all becoming patients. We don't need health insurance, we need lifestyle insurance!

The runaway cost of this is passed right back to us like another tax, and more and more of us can't afford it. You see the headlines: Health costs are dragging America down. Healthcare Leaves Many In Debt. We're bankrupting ourselves, and a healthcare crisis is looming. Is there another way?

There is. Good health is the best and cheapest health insurance. Good health is inexpensive and low-tech. We just have to resolve to have it.

Listen to Ramona, a patient of mine who lost forty pounds, brought her cholesterol down 70 points, and avoided becoming a lifestyle patient: "I want a discount on my health insurance, or I want everyone else to take care of themselves, because I'm paying the price!"

Do the Food Tree and Watch Your Life Transform!

Because I've helped so many diabetic patients in my practice, I recently approached a major HMO and told them that I could help their members with adult onset diabetes. They scoffed: "What? That's impossible. No one can cure diabetes." We don't have to "cure" diabetes, we can teach people to prevent it, reverse it, and live diabetes-free. Many patients would like to—the sad thing is, they just don't know how. They're shocked when I tell them that this option is available to them. No more medications, no more complications, no more being a patient. We are failing our patients by not encouraging them to help themselves become well.

For ten years I've shown that most cases of diabetes can be reversed in a short time. When my patients eat healthily, get off their medication, and take a nice vacation with the money they would have spent on medication, it's very gratifying.

Medication or vacation—which would you rather have?

One pill cuts the sugar, another thins the blood, and a third one makes you happy.

This doesn't sound like fun.

It's much faster and easier to treat symptoms. Partly driven by the pharmaceutical industry, doctors are trained to approach your problem by prescribing medication after medication. Nutrition gets in the way of the patient numbers and sales volume! According to their doctrine, we should really work to get everyone on at least one medication—at least a measly statin! The easiest way to do this is to lower the treatment criteria for all metabolic diseases, and this is exactly what has happened. If we do our research on overweight, unstable patients, it's easy to show that lowering one parameter dramatically is better than not lowering any at all. Let's look through their lens for a minute: Though I'm a thin, active nonsmoker, I now need at least a blood pressure medication, despite the fact that my blood pressure has been normal and stable for as long as I can remember. If they found out that there was diabetes in my family I'd be a lifestyle patient and a statistic on their best-selling drug list! Point: research should be done on groups of well people like me to determine whether or not I need medications.

Have you seen the list of the twenty best-selling drugs? You're probably taking one of them. The first six are all remedies against bad eating—to the tune of nearly $10 billion a year.

In the face of all the information available, this seems medieval to me. I'm keeping my body normal and avoiding doctors. I firmly believe you deserve a chance to do the same. It's my duty to explain what's really wrong with you and give you a chance to help yourself. This way, you at least know the alternative is there. The list of reasons to visit your doctor escalates with every pound you gain, as does your medication list. The medico-pharmaceutical complex wants you!

Did you know that for every pound you gain, you put four pounds of pressure on your joints? So when you lose one pound, you take four pounds of pressure off your knees and hips. This information, combined with what you read here, could save you a lot of pain! For every pound you gain, you're asking for diabetes. For each pound you lose, you reduce your risk by some 4%.

Created in the image of Frankenstein's Monster?

We have been so misled and blind sided that we have abandoned the idea of good health altogether We define high cholesterol as lack of statins and high blood sugar as lack of the latest pills or injections. As long as we keep thinking this way there is no way out.

Here's the classic patient with elevated blood pressure, who's given a diuretic for it, which unmasks latent diabetes. Now the patient needs medication for diabetes. His cholesterol is a little high? Add a statin. Joint pain? Add an anti-inflammatory, which may produce stomach-acid problems. Add the antacid. Now the patient really feels sick, and probably feels miserable too. No problem, bring on the antidepressants. You can imagine this patient might be in need of a little Viagra by now.

This poor patient staggers around like Frankenstein's monster, stitched together by sugar and prescription drugs, while we wait for the next wonder drug—the one that will conquer it all. We're now beginning to see "polypills" that contains all these medications rolled into one. And none of it had to be.

Lynn came to me weighing 280 pounds and on all the diabetes medications she could take, including 70 units of insulin. She now suffered from too much insulin, or hyperinsulinemia, in itself a medical problem. She had gained ten pounds, was bloated, hungry, tired, and almost unable to walk. She dropped ten pounds and came off most of the insulin in three weeks. She now goes to gym and loves it. "Amazing," her doctor said. No, not really—just biochemistry. And it works every time. In research language this is called reproducible results.

Good News—It's Not Your Parents' Fault!

Jim's cholesterol level was 235. His doctor told Jim that he had picked "bad family genes" and prescribed a statin. The doctor neglected to point out that Jim was forty pounds overweight and lived on sugar and beer! True, Jim's parents had passed their eating habits on to him, and this was the result. But before long, the Food Tree cured Jim's "bad genes."

You may have heard about how hopeless you are if you don't take advantage of the wonder drugs. Yet the knowledge you need is still kept from you. Because you don't yet know any better, you sit there and think that your "bad genes" will kill you. Don't believe it. By the end of this book, you'll have all the tools you need to take back your health.

Bad News—It's Your Grandparents' Fault!

Well, don't laugh! Let's peek into the future of epigenetics: It proposes that the environment partly regulates how genes express themselves. Pembrey and Bygren have done work suggesting nutrition as a regulator. That means your grandfather's eating habits could modify his own genes thereby influencing how you eat!

The message is: Looking at our current state of weight and health, what are we passing on to our children?

Jane, a Patient Transformed by the Food Tree

I will never forget Jane, who became my patient some years ago. She had gained weight after a foot injury. This had raised her blood sugar, which in turn brought on diabetes. As she graduated through all the medications, including insulin, she kept gaining weight—which caused high blood pressure and indigestion. Jane's doctor added a blood pressure medication and an acid blocker. Her foot was now causing her more pain.

When Jane started having an irritable bladder, she was given a medication that caused dry mouth. By then, Jane weighed 280 pounds and felt terrible about herself, so her doctor prescribed an antidepressant. This mixture of medications didn't agree with her. She appeared in my office, dazed and disheveled and crying, repeating, "I'm so depressed because I'm so sick!"

I started her on a health-restoring weight loss program. She came back in one week a transformed person, well dressed and groomed, and well spoken. She explained, "I'm actually quite eloquent!"

Within a week Jane was able to taper off her insulin. As her meticulously charted blood sugars approached normal, she gradually stopped her other diabetes medications. I could hardly believe she was the same person who had stumbled into my office.

After three weeks, she stopped taking the acid blocker and the antidepressant. She then stopped the bladder medication, because her bladder was just fine.

One day, she came back a little disappointed. She had seen her internist, who predicted skeptically, "You'll start eating badly again, and then you'll be back!"

Jane lost fifty pounds in six months and was off her blood pressure medication. In addition, her foot pain, the original cause of her first doctor visit, was gone. At that point, she had to move away due to a family problem. From a note she sent me: "Your wonderful program saved my life!" Go for it, Jane! You and other patients like you are living testimony to the benefits of good nutrition. Wherever you are, I hope you're finding the strength to stay well.

Medications treat the symptoms, but the underlying disease marches on. *Only* nutrition can reverse metabolic illnesses. My fellow physicians ignore this or scoff at it. The only doctors who freely advertise weight loss as a remedy for metabolic illnesses are bariatric (weight loss) surgeons. Unfortunately, complications from bariatric surgery, such as malabsorption and deficiency disorders, still leave the patient a patient. The long-term healthcare costs for bariatric surgery patients are about the same as for those who remain obese. Overweight ill people were once well. Perhaps they had a few pounds to lose. In a different world, they would not have become medicinal Frankensteins or candidates for surgery. We are creating our own reality, and we are ticking time bombs!

CHAPTER 3
Lower Your Weight Setpoint

In order to understand the Food Tree, you need to sort out what food is and how it interacts with your body. Only then will you able to take control of your weight by lowering the thermostat that determines your weight setpoint.

Body Composition

Your body can roughly be divided into two components: lean body and fat. Your lean body, that is, your muscle, heart, lungs, and other vital organs, even your blood cells, are made of protein. The other component, fat, is your insulation layer. Some of us may be low on muscle mass if we haven't eaten adequate protein, but most of us have too much of the fat component. The level of body fat considered optimal for women is 17%, for men 22%. Because this is a difficult measurement, an easier estimate has been invented for use as a general guideline.

Body Mass Index

To roughly measure your body composition, we use a calculation based on the ratio of lean body mass to fat called the body mass index, or BMI, which is derived from this formula: weight in kilograms divided by height in meters, squared. Use the chart on page 116 to calculate your own BMI. The Web site of the National Heart, Lung, and Blood Institute, www.nhlbisupport.com/bmi/, also gives you these tables. When your BMI is stable at around 22, your lean body to fat proportion is about right for good health. Your metabolism is working smoothly—you probably eat well and feel good in general.

Note: The BMI calculations are based on the average man or woman, who might not eat adequate protein or get enough exercise to maintain muscle mass. In a balanced program such as the Food Tree, you would be a smaller size at a slightly higher weight, because you'd have optimal muscle mass, and muscle is heavier than fat. Men, due to their greater muscle mass, typically have a higher BMI than women of the same height. Tall, muscular, well-proportioned men often end up at a BMI just below 25, while the table favors small women.

BMI and Obesity

So if your BMI is around 22—great! You're probably eating right for your health. If, however, your BMI is 25 or above, you are in the beginning stages of metabolic illness and should curb it right now— you may be compromising your health and putting yourself at risk for eventual problems.

Resetting Your Weight Thermostat

Your body has several internal thermostats that regulate hunger, weight, and health. Hunger/satiety is very complicated—some of it is beyond the scope of this book. The following basic components are included in your weight thermostat, which you deal with on a daily basis when you eat.

Stomach Hunger

When you feel an empty, gnawing feeling from not eating enough, that may be stomach hunger for lack of volume. Eating adequate fiber is very important in turning off your stomach-volume hunger without consuming unnecessary calories. More on fiber in chapter 4.

Brain Transmitter Substance-related Hunger and Satiety

A host of brain transmitter substances affect your weight. The best-known ones are serotonin and noradrenalin. They also influence your mood, energy, and even migraines. We see this among patients who, taking serotonin-active drugs for depression or headaches, lose or gain weight. The very complicated relationship between these compounds is beyond the scope of this book.

We can't show changes in the blood or brain level of these substances with what we eat. What we can show is an indirect effect. Good nutrition has a stabilizing effect on mood and can lessen or cure migraines, depression, and other mood disorders. It also makes you feel full! Appetite suppressants influence these brain transmitter substances to regulate your hunger. The now-infamous Fen-Phen was an example of that. A series of newly discovered weight-related hormones are being studied in hope of finding new obesity drugs.

The problem with using medications to lose weight is that they won't teach you what's going wrong—nor will they allow you to work with the regulatory mechanisms your body makes available to you. They simply make you feel full, even if your blood sugar is low and your stomach empty. They obliterate your body's own efforts to protect its lean body mass. You may stop eating and lose weight fast, including muscle mass, but when you stop taking the appetite suppressant, your appetite goes back to where it was, and your struggle with food and weight continues.

It's also possible to alter these brain-mechanism levels through surgery, but that's not a realistic option. Fortunately, good nutrition works the same way—it stabilizes mood and makes you feel full.

Insulin—The Master Regulator

The most important regulator is the one you deal with daily when you eat: your friend, foe, and master switch for all things metabolic, the major anabolic hormone insulin.

Understanding insulin is key to controlling your weight because insulin determines most things in your body, including your weight and health, and *you* determine the amount of insulin your body produces. We used to think insulin simply regulated our blood sugar—a gross underestimation. Insulin determines sugar regulation, the production and breakdown of almost every substance in your body, transportation, storage, and hunger. In short, it determines your cell growth and metabolic state of health. It does so not by itself, but by regulating most other hormones and messengers in the body. Insulin is made in your pancreas and is transported to your cells by your bloodstream.

Insulin is made in response to eating sugar, and sugar only. This is key.

Sugar and Insulin—The Glucose-Insulin Curve

As you go about your day and eat three meals on the Food Tree program, your food intake and insulin production form a curve over time.

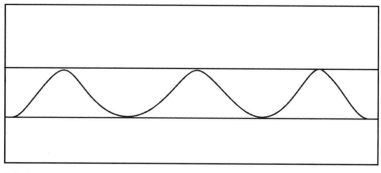

Maintenance:
Three Balanced Meals Per Day

This curve, known as the glucose-insulin curve, works like a thermostat. It regulates your weight, and the top of the curve after a meal defines your *weight setpoint.* It adjusts up or down at any time, depending on the composition of your meal.

When you eat sugar, your blood sugar rises and your pancreas makes insulin—causing your glucose-insulin curve to rise. As the slope and height of the curve increase, so does the setpoint. Insulin transports the sugar from your bloodstream to your cells and, depending on how much energy you need, uses it as energy or stores it as fat. When the process is complete, sugar and insulin return to baseline, repeating at the next meal.

The Glucose-Insulin Window

When you eat three balanced meals a day and expend all the energy you take in, the glucose-insulin curve gently rolls along within the frames shown above, and your setpoint is stable. I refer to this as the *glucose-insulin window.* This is the window you must stay in to maintain your weight.

Note: The glucose-insulin curve is not a numerical blood-sugar curve, but a visualization, a stylized representation, of a biochemical process. For a more detailed curve, see Last et al., *American Family Physician,* vol. 73, #11, June 1, 2006.

A balanced meal triggers a moderate amount of insulin, causing your sugar-insulin curve to rise gently to the upper frame of the window.

In this case, everything you ate is used as energy. Your weight stays the same. As the sugar enters the cell, your blood sugar starts gently dropping, and your insulin production wanes. When your blood sugar reaches the lower frame, you become hungry and repeat the curve. The cycle from fullness to hunger takes four hours or so.

As you might imagine, the slope and height of the curve depends on how much sugar you take in. Can we measure that? We can—though indirectly—with the glycemic index, or GI. This is a scale expressing the effect of various sugars on the curve. It's explained in chapter 4, and the GI table starting on page 121.

You probably noticed the similarity of the names glucose-insulin curve (G-I curve) and the glycemic index (GI). That's no accident, since the glycemic index is largely responsible for the curve. The Food Tree keeps your curve in the window. But when you eat too much refined sugar, the story changes.

Continental Breakfast and the G-I Curve

When you eat a high-sugar meal—a breakfast of bread with jam, or a pastry, for example—your blood sugar rises rapidly, overshooting the upper frame of the window and forcing your pancreas to produce large amounts of insulin to transport all that sugar into the cells. If your body doesn't need all the sugar for energy, it will store the excess as fat, and you'll gain weight.

You feel great from all that sugar—but not for long: as it leaves the bloodstream, your blood sugar levels drop, making you feel very hungry again. The more sugar you take in, the more rapidly your G-I curve drops, and the hungrier you become. You may even develop low blood sugar (hypoglycemia) and become unwell.

You feel weak, tired, and cranky—your G-I curve is below the window—and you need a quick fix to raise your curve. You need pure sugar!

Descent into Addiction

So you find your fix, and when you feed that need for sugar, the vicious cycle repeats. Because you're compelled to eat sugar to raise your ever-sagging blood sugar, this represents a physical addiction curve. The high sugar-insulin curve looks like this:

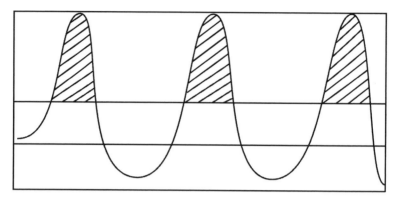

Weight Gain:
Three High Sugar Meals Per Day

What goes down must come up. Two things happen now: your setpoint has moved to the top of this curve, and you're storing what's above the window.

You now understand why people claim to become hungrier all day despite eating breakfast. If you eat a high-sugar breakfast, as opposed to giving your body building blocks that turn off the thermostat, you've revved up your setpoint and end up chasing it all day long.

Weight gain or loss happens at the setpoint, not in between.

Sugar is Addictive!

The message is clear—too much refined sugar is addictive because it causes a steep slalom curve that you cannot stop. The curve never stays in the normal window; it only intersects the normal curve on the way up or down while it keeps you racing between feeling great and feeling cranky—and totally addicted to the next rescue.

If you continue to eat large quantities of sugar, you risk exhausting your pancreas and eventually losing the ability to produce enough insulin to metabolize all the sugar you consume. You become insulin resistant, or pre-diabetic, with the next step being diabetes.

That means diabetes is exhaustion of your pancreas from eating sugar!

Nearly all the patients who come to me can describe this curve perfectly. They can feel the euphoria of the sugar high, and the hunger, fatigue, irritability, and depressed mood of the sugar low.

- *Remember: When your G-I curve is above the window, you are gaining weight!*

Your Hunger Thermostat and Sugar Addiction

The more refined sugar you eat, the higher you drive your hunger thermostat, forever setting your weight point higher. You may have heard that if you drink one less can of soda a day you'll lose around fifteen pounds in a year. Unfortunately, once you need that sugar to feed this curve, you'll find a sugary substitute for that can of soda.

You now see that once you've been on this addiction curve, you're only one large dose of sugar away from it at all times!

Switching Sugar of Choice

Laura told me, "I'm addicted to coffee." She couldn't see that she was actually addicted to sugar-laced coffee drinks. Realizing that they wouldn't work for weight loss, she substituted smoothies for coffee drinks, which, at the equivalent of up to twelve tablespoons of sugar per serving, were no bargain for her poor pancreas! She soon found a new substitute: corn. Good try, but still a high GI choice.

Cutting Calories Is Not the Answer!

You might resort to dieting the curve down by cutting calories. You might spend your allotted calories on sugar based "non-foods" which will deprive you of essential foodstuffs. This will produce hunger simply because you're not feeding your body what it needs. The next type of dieter is "the hero," who doesn't eat all day. This relates especially to the person who eats one meal a day and gains weight. Nearly 90 percent of my patients fall into this category.

No breakfast, poor or no lunch—great intentions that fall apart at dinner and later. Sound familiar?

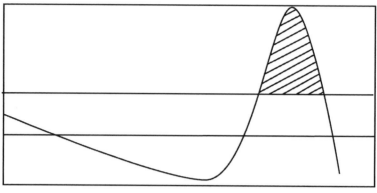

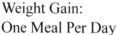

Weight Gain:
One Meal Per Day

Individuals on this curve are spiraling downward most of the day. Their blood sugar is very depleted, which causes ravenous hunger. By dinner, they eat an enormous meal to make up for all the deprivation.

The area under the curve, the whole load of that one meal, is way above the G-I window. No matter how much these people starve during the day, they overcompensate by eating too much of everything at night, and their body stores it as fat. This curve also explains why appetite-suppressant medications do not work.

It also explains why long-term weight maintenance is so difficult. Once you've lived on the addiction curve, your body wants to go back there. It might not take much sugar to get your insulin production going. This is why I see patients who don't stay with me in weight maintenance regain their weight.

Drugs Fool Your Brain Thermostat—But Not the G-I Curve

As we said, appetite suppressant medications change the mood/serotonin/norepinephrine levels in your brain, blocking the hunger signals sent by the G-I curve and your blood sugar. If you take these medications and stop eating, your blood sugar plunges, but your brain says you're full and feel great. You fail to eat enough, and in balance, and you lose lean body mass. As soon as you stop taking the medication, your angry body reclaims lost muscle—along with equal amounts of fat.

When your body comes back from this type of deficiency, you tend to overeat to make up for lost time. You get on one of the weight-gain curves shown above, and end up at a higher weight. This is called weight cycling.

Break the Cycle with the Food Tree

So how do you get off the addiction curve? Learning what sugar really is, and how it affects your blood chemistry, is the first step toward taking control of your weight and your life. Now that you understand how sugar affects your weight, you can begin to appreciate the power of the Food Tree. Let's look at the sugar-insulin curve of a person on the Food Tree, in the weight-loss mode.

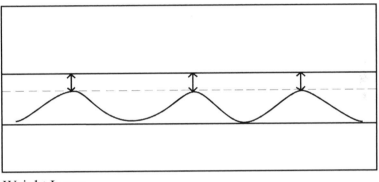

Weight Loss:
Three Meals Per Day

As you can see, the G-I curve does not reach the upper frame of the window. The less sugar you eat, the less insulin you produce, and the less the curve rises. Remember that weight loss, just like weight gain, happens after you eat, at the setpoint. The distance between the top of your glucose-insulin curve (called the postprandial blood-sugar load) and the upper frame of the window represents your weight loss. If you added a snack in the two mild troughs of the weight-loss curve, it would look like this:

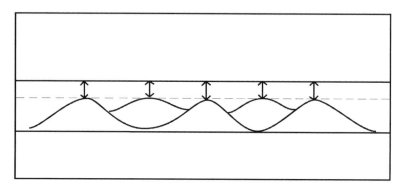

Weight Loss:
Three Meals And Two Snacks Per Day

Between the setpoint and the upper frame of the window, this curve shows a constant space that represents weight loss. It also shows that this curve keeps your blood sugar nearly even throughout the day. Best of all, you lose weight while feeling full. This is the Food Tree.

The Glycemic Index—Adjusting Your Body's Thermostat or Setpoint

All these curves demonstrate that you determine your weight setpoint with sugar. Every time you eat, you adjust your weight thermostat by setting your G-I curve in or out of the window. The amount of sugar you eat, and what kind, determines where your setpoint tops out.

The effect of the sugar you eat on the G-I curve is your adjustable weight thermostat. Metabolic health, mood, hunger, and energy follow this curve.

Give Your Pancreas a Break!

Remember: Type 2 diabetes is a result of having eaten enough sugar to exhaust your pancreas' ability to produce insulin in response to all this sugar. This is similar to abusing cousin alcohol. The treatment is to stop consuming the toxin.

When you take anti-diabetic tablets, you push your exhausted pancreas to produce more insulin, and it will eventually fail. When you start insulin, you create hyperinsulinemia, a condition marked by bloating, weight gain, fatigue, and continued inflammation.

If you remove the sugar instead, you take the pressure off your pancreas to produce insulin because the flow of sugar into the cells is brought into the normal window. You can now understand that anything that raises your G-I curve above the window is not a food, but a toxin that destroys your pancreas and causes inflammation and addiction. And the treatment is to stop the destructive process.

In this chapter, I've described how your body's weight thermostat regulates weight and how it affects the glucose-insulin curve. In summary:

- Your glucose-insulin curve is your metabolic health and weight thermostat.
- The top of the curve is your weight setpoint.
- This is the scientific basis behind the Food Tree.

Balancing Your Nutrition with the Food Tree

When you eat with the Food Tree, your setpoint is where you want it and your G-I curve is beautifully in the window. You can feel it. Your mood, energy, and hunger level are now all on an even keel. If you don't have excess amounts of insulin, you can't store sugar as fat. This is, in part, what the Atkins and other high-protein programs are based on. As you remove sugar, your body needs other nutrients to keep your blood-sugar level even.

Eating adequate protein is key to maintaining good muscle mass and preventing hunger. It also breaks down slowly into sugar, using energy in the process. It also triggers a beneficial hormone called glucagon. This is the counter-regulatory hormone to insulin, and is your second safety valve against low blood sugar. In addition to keeping your blood sugar from getting too low, glucagon puts your body into breakdown mode (catabolic state) as opposed to storage mode (anabolic state), which means that whatever you eat after you've raised your glucagon will tend to be broken down rather than stored. You increase your glucagon production by eating protein. This also helps break your sugar addiction.

The basic formula for nutrition is the balance between driving your G-I curve up with sugar and down with protein.

Sugar →Raised G-I curve → Weight gain, hunger, bad health
Protein → Lowered G-I curve → Weight loss, fullness, good health

You now see that you don't need a "diet" or anything else—you simply need to understand this basic formula and what you're eating. Then you'll know which way you are driving your curve.

But there is more to balanced nutrition: fiber addresses the volume-related hunger mechanism and slows down absorption. If our fiber intake is low, we need to eat more of the other components to become full, skewing the balance. Bulk is beautiful! See the discussion of fiber in chapter 4.

What About Fat?

Fat is crucial to good health. It's vital that you get enough fat—but the right kind of fat. It doesn't impact the G-I curve directly, but it shares one quality with protein and fiber: it stabilizes (that is, lowers) the GI of carbohydrates because it tempers carbohydrate absorption. You'll find a full discussion of fat as a nutrient in chapter 4.

Some Consequences of What We've Learned So Far

Some people can eat a lot more than others and yet stay the same weight. Why is that? The answer is partly nervous energy, but largely it's in the way their thermostats work. Human traits, including insulin sensitivity, are distributed on a normal curve, or bell curve, represented here:

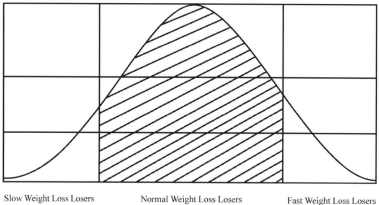

Slow Weight Loss Losers   Normal Weight Loss Losers   Fast Weight Loss Losers

The Normal Population Distribution Curve — (Bell Curve)

The average person of normal weight (some 50–75 percent of us) produces insulin in proportion to the sugar eaten. The persons on the lower end of the curve are very insulin-sensitive; they can eat large amounts of sugar, don't need much insulin to metabolize it, and stay the same weight. Because their insulin production is lower for the same sugar consumption, they don't go into the slalom curve of storage, hypoglycemia, reactive sugar eating, and weight gain. They're the lucky ones who, regardless of what they eat, seem immune to sliding onto the addiction curve. Such normal-weight individuals comprise only about 20 percent of us.

The unlucky individuals at the top of the curve (10–25 percent) need a lot of insulin to metabolize sugar. They gain weight easily, and become diabetic if they keep pushing sugar on their bodies. The good news is that if they keep their sugar intake low, their sugar-insulin curve and their weight stay normal. Again, because we're dealing with an addiction curve, this explains the very small number of people who keep their weight off in the long term. They're only a slip away from the slalom curve. Once back on it, many of them let it run its course until they're back to their old setpoint, and can't explain how they let it happen. Do you recognize something here? At this point, most of us with normal insulin sensitivity eat enough sugar to push our curve into weight gain, and we see more and more pancreas fatigue (insulin resistance).

When you consume protein and fiber-rich, low-GI carbohydrates (hereafter shortened to carbs), your hunger mechanism shuts off. Though fat in the quantities we're talking about here doesn't affect this hunger mechanism appreciably, it's all the more crucial to what happens when we start processing food. This is the essence of the Food Tree.

If you adhere to the Food Tree and still have metabolic abnormalities, you're part of the population that has a particularly strong genetic predisposition for certain conditions, and you should be treated for it. Even if you fall into this group, if you maintain a normal weight and are otherwise healthy you'll need less medicine and will feel better. Reread the story of my brother Roald (end of chapter 1), which illustrates this point.

But I Need That Sugar for a Quick Pick-me-up

If your energy is always sagging but returns after eating sugar, you just got busted! You aren't eating enough food for your body to keep up its energy. You're patching with sugar and creating an addiction curve.

Why Can't I Just Take a Pill?

You can, but statistics aren't in your favor. I've already shown you one reason why taking medication isn't the best way to go. Here's another:

Good nutrition reduces your health risk twofold compared with taking pills. When you take pills for diabetes, blood pressure, cholesterol, etc., you're covering up different manifestations of bad eating with pills. The underlying inflammatory reaction in your body caused by bad nutrition marches on, and might find new ways to express itself. You can also see that if you take a weight-reducing drug, you're not really working with your body. You might end up losing lean body mass, and, as so many of you know, the weight tends to come back when you stop taking the drug.

Is Bariatric Surgery an Option?

Unheard of some thirty years ago, bariatric surgery is mushrooming like the obesity epidemic itself. Most people find it daunting to lose 100-plus pounds. Bariatric surgery aligns the patient with the very culture that created the problem. He or she can eat sugar, though it becomes self-limiting because it's not well tolerated. Until we change the environment that creates these patients, we're stuck with the results. It's a sad testimony to our failure as a culture.

How Fast Can I Lose Weight with the Food Tree?

We've all seen the ads: "Lose five pounds a week!" That, of course, is like "Get rich in two months with our wealth seminar." The average body can lose six to ten pounds per month, depending on several conditions:

- The genetic type of weight loser you are (some people simply can take off the pounds faster—the rate of weight loss *is based on genetic factors*);
- *How much you lower your G-I curve;*
- *How much energy you burn by activity.*

Activity influences things more profoundly than you might think. It lowers your entire G-I curve, thereby lowering your setpoint. It's so important for you to understand this fact that I've devoted chapter 8 to it.

The point here is that the speed of weight loss doesn't matter. What matters is that you start giving your poor, neglected body the building blocks it needs, rather than inundating and poisoning it with garbage, and put yourself on the road to good health. You'll feel thin long before you become thin. There's no substitute for feeling in control.

Dump This Advice

Many of my patients who want to lose five pounds are told by their doctors, "You don't have a weight problem." Wrong. *One pound over normal weight is overweight!* Because of the progressive nature of weight gain, this is so. Whether you need to lose one pound or a hundred pounds, you have a problem if you can't lose that weight.

When doctors see patients at the beginning stages of weight gain, they do them no favors by waiting to address the problem. They fail the patient right there. The longer they wait, the bigger the problem grows, and the harder it is to turn around. I'm happy to teach people maintenance, so they can end their struggle before it becomes a problem.

Until we accept scientific reasoning and teach people to keep the G-I curve in the window, we remain willing victims perennially searching for the next miracle.

Feel Great with the Food Tree!

Almost every patient who has come off the physical addiction curve and normalized their G-I curve is astounded by how good they feel in a matter of days. Bloating and edema disappear, blood sugar and blood pressure drop, and energy soars. After two weeks on my program, Ann said, "I used to crash at nine p.m. I now have so much energy I'm up cleaning my house at eleven. My depression is gone. I feel wonderful!"

In this chapter, you learned the scientific framework behind the Food Tree. In the next, we'll examine the elements of healthy eating, and teach you how to keep your G-I curve in the window by designing your own personal Food Tree.

CHAPTER 4
Introducing Nutrition—What's in the Food Tree?

This chapter introduces the nutritional concepts crucial to building your Food Tree. Our bodies recognize the following sources of calories, also called macronutrients (large): protein, fat, carbohydrates, and alcohol. Leaving out alcohol, the others are the three basic food groups. Good health also depends on fiber and water. Let's start by looking at the true nature of carbohydrates, also known as sugar. We've explained that some carbohydrates are food and some are toxins. The distinction happens on a sliding scale, and depends on which carbs and how much of them you eat.

All carbohydrates are variations of the basic sugar molecule called glucose. With slight variations, glucose takes the form of malt sugar, milk sugar, or fruit sugars, which are linked together differently to give them different names and chemical characteristics.

The difference between the useful carbs and the damaging sugars is, therefore, a biochemical one. The glucose molecules found in complex carbohydrates are more tightly bound, and require more time and effort for your body to free the sugar and thus raise your blood sugar. Simple refined sugar molecules require your body to do almost no work to raise your blood sugar.

Sugar—The Sliding GI Slope to Bad Health

To conquer sugar, you need to know its true nature on the scale from toxin to food. Otherwise, you'll find yourself on a slippery slope to bad health. This scale is called the *glycemic index, or GI scale.* It assigns a relative number to the rate of absorption and thus the rise in blood sugar when you eat enough of any carb to derive 50 grams of sugar (equivalent to nearly two ounces, or three tablespoons). The GI describes how fast and hard your pancreas has to work to produce insulin in response.

The sugar power of glucose is given the top rating, 100. Fiber rates 0, because it's not absorbable. Below is a representation of the scale of carbohydrates from bad (100) to good (0). The bad simple carbohydrates on the left side have little or no nutritional value. GI decreases as you move to the right on this scale, but note how the nutritional value increases.

Sugar > grain products > potatoes > corn/rice > fruits > legumes > vegetables > fiber
100_____0

As we move to the right of the scale, the carbohydrates are bound together more tightly. The tighter the binding, the slower your blood sugar rises. Although they're a type of sugar, the most complex carbohydrates, called fiber, have such complex bonding that we can't absorb them, and they remain in the gastrointestinal tract as bulk.

As you can see, sugars and grains are easy for your body to process—too easy. In reality, they're a deadly pair, quickly raising your blood sugar and insulin to unhealthy levels. Rice, potatoes, and corn are fairly rapid inducers of insulin also. The more refined and cooked, the faster they work. As the scale shifts to the right, carbohydrates are made up of more tightly bound glucose molecules that take your body longer to unravel and raise your blood sugar. The farther to the right of this curve you eat, the slower your blood sugar rises, the gentler the rise of your insulin, and the more food value. To the far right we have fiber, which we need for the stomach and colon to feel full and function well.

GI Matters

On this scale, pure glucose tops out at 100. This means that if you eat enough sugar to get 50 grams of glucose, your GI tops the scale at 100. Table sugar is half fructose (GI 23), which lowers its GI for 50 grams to 70. Some scales are based on white bread being 100. That should tell you the true story—white bread is nothing but sugar. On the other hand, the glycemic index of vegetables and legumes is low, and this is the end of the scale you mainly should be on. You'll find the information and the glycemic index chart starting on page 121.

Size Matters!

You don't eat 50 grams of pure sugar each time you eat carbohydrates, so how do you know the GI of what you've eaten? The GI of carbohydrates is linear and in proportion to how much you eat. The portion size that gives you 50 grams of sugar varies greatly from carb to carb. This is critical to understanding GI.

For that reason the nutritional guide starting on page 121 is annotated to give you the GI of the most common carbs.

For example, it takes some 50 grams (three tablespoons) of table sugar, but three slices of bread (on average) to reach GI 70. One tablespoon of sugar and/or slice of bread would have one third of full 70, which is 23. It would take half a pound of potatoes, but almost two pounds of apples, to reach GI 70. Finally, for most vegetables, it's almost impossible to eat yourself above a nice, safe, low GI in the 20s. Size really matters!

Type Matters!

Fructose has GI 23; that is, three tablespoons (50 grams) gives you GI 23, as opposed to the GI 70 of three tablespoons of table sugar. A tablespoon would yield about one-third or 8. Fructose was used as an alternative sugar for diabetics before the very low-calorie and non-caloric sweeteners gained popular use. The reported evil of fructose comes from the myth that it causes liver damage. If you consider that our greatest source (50 percent) of fructose is table sugar, that would be a lot of damaged livers! The other problem is its extensive use in processed foods as "high fructose corn syrup," the new pariah of anti-fructose crusaders. The truth is that corn syrup has the same composition as table sugar and honey, "high fructose" or not. The problem is the same as for sugar: overuse.

We know that size matters. Now you see that type matters as well. Some fruits have more glucose and less fructose, and some are more fibrous. This changes the GI. Grain types show the same kind of variation. These variations are relatively small. If you mash, juice, or cook carbs, GI goes up. The change is dramatic in carrots, which have GI 30 in raw form and 85 cooked. In both cases, though, you'd have to eat two pounds to get there. The less you cook carrots, the better. Grains are interesting, in that whole grain has low GI. For instance, whole barley has GI 22. Mill it to make bread, and its GI can go as high as 70, depending on the milling.

Low-GI Carbs—A Brilliant Idea for Your Health

When you examine the Food Tree, you'll see that the large lower branches are the most important carbs in your diet. Our main source of dietary fiber comes from low-GI carbohydrates. Mostly vegetables legumes and berries, these carbs contain vitamins and trace minerals. The brilliance of their color hides some 4,000 micronutrients called polyphenols or flavonoids. Polyphenols are antioxidant, anti-aging agents. Immune boosters as well, they protect us from cancer and other illnesses. The more color a vegetable has, the more polyphenols it contains. These carbs are nutrient dense, as opposed to sugar, which is primarily calorie dense.

Fiber—the Fabulous Fabric of Food

As you have seen, fiber is a major player in the nutritional formula. It is an important GI stabilizer and supplies the volume needed to keep our intestines healthy. But it has another major function: It lowers our bad cholesterol (LDL) by trapping it as it enters the intestine from the liver— no small job description for something you might not even be paying attention to. And it is the bulk that makes you feel full on fewer calories. The so-called water-soluble type of fiber is the most effective for lowering cholesterol. It's found in oat bran, legumes, apples, pears, citrus fruits, berries, and nuts. Peas, beans, and squash are high fiber and low GI and are great choices. Fiber and protein in balance are the basics of fullness and wellness, and both loom large on the Food Tree. The insoluble or bulk ones are found in other grains, seeds, carrots, cucumbers, zucchini, celery, and other vegetables. You can see why I don't recommend juices or milled grains—they supply more sugar and less fiber.

The Higher, the More Toxic

The low-GI carbohydrates are the unfermented equivalents of naturally occurring alcohols. It takes a lot to get drunk!

The medium-GI carbs are comparable to wine. They're fine in moderation, but high doses will harm you. A drink or a serving of dark bread will not harm you, but a bottle of wine or a loaf of bread will put your blood sugar in the gutter. Pure sugar is as toxic to you as pure alcohol, though they metabolize differently.

As we move into the high-GI carbs, the nutritional value plummets as toxic properties increase. They become aggressive, toxic additives, just like cousin alcohol.

What Is a High-GI Carbohydrate?

From what you've learned so far, you now understand that the lower you keep your GI and your blood sugar, the farther you are from activating the inflammatory chain in your body. We call GI 40–50 medium; 50 is definitely high!

A Complex Carb is Not a Complex Carb. Bread Is Not a Staple!

The Food Pyramid and the carb gurus would have you believe that grain products are complex carbs. They are not. They're sugars, some of them more refined than sugar (see the GI for the average cereal in the GI table starting on page 121). Bread as we know it is therefore not a staple food—*it is an additive.* Finely ground flours, rice, potatoes, corn, and cereals are all in this group. Even commercially available whole-grain bread is mostly white flour, with a handful of coarsely ground or whole grain sprinkled in, and made with plenty of honey or other sugar. Scandinavians use darker, coarser flour. The bread I grew up with in Scandinavia is full of fiber and isn't sweet. Oat bread has the lowest glycemic index, which, at around 48, borders on high. Bread was fine when we did physical work; now we're mostly sedentary, which changes the equation.

I've included my mother's recipe for oat bread in the appendices. The coarser the flour, the less the dough sticks together, and it doesn't rise as much as white bread. You may have to practice a little before you get it right. Give it a try—you might enjoy its texture and chewiness.

Do Refined Sugars Have a Use?

Just as small amounts of alcohol are established as a cardiovascular health benefit, sugar has its place in nutrition. Refined sugar delivers one thing: quick, pure, cheap energy. Sugar is our main source of quick energy when we're highly active. We have a predictable adaptation mechanism: exercise burns off sugar quickly, preventing the high blood-sugar peaks and lowering our insulin requirements. The harder we work, the lower the G-I curve.

Excavations in Egypt show that workers had an excellent baseline diet of protein and fat, but it took a lot of bread to roll those two ton blocks of stone up a pyramid. Our ancestors had to run faster than their dinner, and they didn't have bread; they did it all on fruit and honey. Bread just allows for more cheap energy. The problem is that few of us engage in that type of vigorous physical activity nowadays. Even physical laborers in our culture get diabetes when they eat too much sugar.

Traditional European food, including very coarse-grained breads, is the diet of physical laborers. We simply don't work hard enough to need all that fast energy, but we eat as though we do.

We now know that athletes don't need to pasta-load to run a marathon. In fact, if pasta is eaten the night before, the liver has turned it into fat by the next morning, which can make a runner sluggish. Fruit and fruit juices right before exercise will yield the same energy. They'll also supply potassium, magnesium, calcium, and other vital nutrients.

On our Web site, you can meet Ken Newman (his real name), an actor and triathlete who used to carbo-load the night before a race. He now follows our basic athletes' program and sugar-loads before and during the race instead. This has turned him into an amazing winner.

The GI Plot Thickens

I referred to fiber as a glycemic-index stabilizer. Protein and fat work the same way. This means that when eaten together, the protein and fat compete for absorption, thereby lowering GI. Some foods have these stabilizers built in: pasta, chocolate, milk products, ice cream, and nuts. So do pizza, chips, burgers, and fries, but be aware that their lowered GI is outweighed by their high fat content—sometimes really bad fat, which will offset any benefit of the lowered GI.

A Calorie Is Not a Calorie

You've probably heard that a calorie is a calorie. You've now seen that nothing could be further from the truth as far as your body is concerned. The final GI of what you eat determines whether you're feeding the inflammatory chain in your body. Nonfood calories stoke the chain much more quickly than food calories. Low-GI carbs have food value and are generally *nutrient dense*. The nonfood carbohydrates are generally *calorie dense* and have little or no food value.

GI of a Typical Breakfast
2 teaspoons sugar in your coffee (GI 14).
1 slice bread (GI 23).
1 tablespoon jam (GI 17).
Total GI: 54 (high GI, no nutrition).
*Your pancreas is working hard to produce insulin,
and what goes up must come down!*

A Day on the Roller Coaster

When we start the day with refined sugars, we start an insulin roller-coaster ride that lasts all day.

Starting with a Bad Breakfast

At two pieces of toast with jam, our GI skyrockets to $40 + 40 = 80$. Sugar in the coffee adds up quickly. Before we know it, our GI is over 100—off the charts, and the day has only begun!

Moving On to a Bad Lunch

A couple of hours later we're really cranky and hungry again. For lunch we grab a slice of pizza or a sandwich with chips (mostly sugar and bad fat), and the roller coaster continues.

Finishing with the Disaster Dinner

For dinner, try a pasta dish topped off with a piece of cake. Your body is now weeping and wishing it were back in the days of hunting and gathering, when the menu was game, fish, fruit, and berries.

Health Goes Out the G-I Window!

Imagine what happens to your G-I curve when you keep eating this way. You send it out the window, leaving you stuck on the toxic slalom course. Your body is simply not set up to process this stuff. It can deal with it only in small doses, used as an additive, not as food. You are cultivating a garbage tree!

Note: Almost all the metabolic toxins are refined and processed.

Controlling Your GI with the Food Tree

Luckily for us, we can eat within the G-I window with the Food Tree. Our body rewards us with good health when we eat well—and it's so simple! The next chapter provides the details. Until then, here's a preview of breakfast, Food Tree style!

GI of the Food Tree Breakfast

Coffee with no sugar (GI 0).

Yogurt (GI 30 for a quart—GI 7 for 8 oz., one cup, a fourth of a quart); add 2 tablespoons cottage cheese (no GI) to bring your protein count to 15 grams.

1 piece of fruit (GI 10).

Total GI: 17, as opposed to 51!

Alternatively, 3 egg whites will yield your 15 grams of protein at GI 0.

The nutritional value of the Food Tree breakfast is high and the GI load low. You may be wondering how you'll learn to calculate the GI of your foods. It seems complicated, but it's pretty simple as long as you stay away from processed foods. Your nutrition guide starting on page 121 lists the approximate GI of most carb-containing foods.

Eating In the Right Neighborhood

By now you probably realize that the GI table isn't meant to be a precise measurement. It should be used to discern the GI "neighborhood," that is, high, low, or medium.

You don't have to tote around your scale and your laptop. Use the GI table as a rough guide to carbs. A working knowledge of the GI area you're in is all you need, because GI is only an approximate measure to begin with. The GI of a carbohydrate is influenced by its botanical properties (the percentage of certain starches in grains), particle size (a measure of milling, cooking, mashing, or other refinement), absorption (what foods you eat with it), and concentration (juices, for instance). That's why GI has been discredited as a standard of gauging the effect on the body of the carbs we eat. But this is propaganda. GI is very useful when you eat real foods. If you don't, all bets are off anyway.

Eating Is Simple—Stay in the Low-GI Range

First, we shouldn't be eating stuff that's too complicated to assess for GI—it's usually toxic and/or worthless as nutrition. Second, when you mix the carbs with protein and the right fats on the Food Tree, remember they have a stabilizing effect on your GI. Third, this isn't all about numbers, but about assembling your Food Tree to stay in the low range.

I've spent all this time on carbohydrates because they run your G-I thermostat. The Food Tree, however, is centered on your body's need for protein.

Protein—the Trunk of the Tree

Protein comes from *protos,* Greek for *first*. It is named this because it's the only nutritional building block capable of repairing lean body mass. The name implies that even the ancient Greeks understood its importance. Just as our G-I thermostat curve is known, our protein requirements have been known for a long time. My family's turn-of-the-century cookbook states that an adult needs a maintenance supply of 1 gram of protein per kilo of body weight per day. Modern studies have confirmed this repeatedly (Phinney, et al.). See protein requirements on page 118 in the appendices.

We're suffering from a case of mistaken identity. We have vilified protein and relegated it to the additive group. We've made it an almost taboo concept in nutrition, and attack its advocates and users without any scientific basis. We've confused protein with sugar and fat—even with cholesterol. Now we're suffering the consequences. Meanwhile, protein is being used fearlessly by athletes and others who rely on it for good nutrition. It's not clear to me what our enmity toward protein is based on, but for the sake of our health, we need to clear up this misunderstanding.

Our lean body (muscle, heart, lungs, and lean tissues) is made up of biologically complete protein, meaning that it contains all twenty amino acids. Nine of these, called essential amino acids, can't be produced by the body, so we must eat them to maintain good health.

In addition, our blood cells, most enzymes, hormones, and other messenger substances of our bodies are also made of this crucial building block. Simply put, our bodies are built on and often communicate in the language of protein.

Sources of Protein

Complete proteins are found mainly in animal products such as meat, fish, poultry, eggs, and dairy, but also in soy products. There is no "bad" animal protein. Most fish, poultry, meat, and cheese have some 20–30 mg of cholesterol per ounce, and varying degrees of saturated fat.

If we choose lean products and eat them within the confines of normal weight, they're all part of a healthy diet.

We get into trouble if we eat high-fat foods and gain weight. Saturated animal fat can contribute to high cholesterol and heart disease. If the meat is lean and grass-fed, the limited fat actually supplies us valuable conjugated linoleic acids (CLA) and the amino acid leucine, as do dairy fats. Both are natural defenses against diabetes and heart disease. Soy products vary in fat content. Milk and yogurt have whey, which contains lactose, and are low-GI dairy carbohydrates as well as proteins. Cheese can be high in saturated fat. Cheeses that crumble easily (feta, for example) are leaner; cheeses that don't (cheddar, for example) are fattier. The creamy cheeses are highest in fat.

The purer the protein product, the more it can be a tool for weight loss if used properly. There are a number of protein products out there such as powders and bars. Some have high fat and sugar content, leaving the protein content low. Protein supplementation is neither good nor bad, and can be a convenient aid to busy people who want to start their day right. It can save you from the pastry or candy bar that destroys your G-I curve immediately, and the high insulin that will start you off to eating more the entire day. It can also be a great snack. I supplement many of my weight-loss programs with complete protein, containing all 20 amino acids. because it's easy for my patients and supplies the required protein without extra calories. My protein drinks are available through my Web site. If you have a particular product that you like, make sure it's a complete protein.

Our bodies are in a constant state of breakdown and repair of protein-based tissues. We have a basic daily requirement of protein that will keep our lean body healthy and fill us so we don't need to chase our hunger mechanism with sugar. If we skimp on protein in our diet during weight loss, we lose muscle and become hungry. Because working muscles burn a lot of energy, muscle loss decreases our metabolic rate and may make it harder to stay at a lower weight.

Daily Protein Requirements

I use the protein requirements for weight loss established by the National Task Force for the Prevention and Treatment of Obesity (*JAMA*, August 1993). These are summarized in the formula on page 118.

Requirements change with activity, athletics, pregnancy, and nursing, as noted in the table. I remind you again: This is not a high-protein diet—it is what your body needs to support muscle in weight loss.

Returning to the myth that too much protein is bad for you, history and research don't support this notion. The Inuit and other Eskimo people have lived for thousands of years on a diet consisting mostly of marine-based fat and protein.

In Alaska and parts of Canada where these cultures live, access to carbohydrates was sporadic and limited mainly to the summer months. The noted Canadian explorer Vilhjalmur Stefansson brought proof of this to America in 1928, voluntarily isolating himself with a colleague for a year in Bellevue Hospital in New York. Under the auspices of the AMA they lived exclusively on 100–140 grams of protein, with the remaining calories coming from fat. Getting enough vitamin C was vital, but he had learned how to obtain it the Inuit way—by eating raw meat. A minimum of vitamins and trace minerals can be gleaned from meat and fish. He also proved that fiber and polyphenols are not essential—apparently, we can live without them. They are, therefore, not designated as vitamins, but that should not be an excuse for shunning them and living on the edge.

Recently, Layman's series of scientific studies on high-protein diets confirmed the above observations. Doctors used to tell patients with kidney damage to restrict their protein. That's not necessarily the case anymore. Nephrologists have changed their view; for the most part, they now allow unrestricted protein in patients' diets. If you have diabetic or any other form of kidney damage, you should follow the nutritional program your doctor sets up for you.

Protein Works Biochemical Wonders

Proteins don't have a glycemic index, which means that they don't raise insulin enough to register on the GI scale. In fact, quite the opposite happens: protein stabilizes GI by slowing the absorption of any carb you eat with it. As noted earlier, protein triggers the release of glucagon, the counter-regulatory hormone to insulin. Glucagon keeps your blood sugar from falling too low, and speeds up fat burning by triggering the production of ketone bodies from fat, which are burned off as fuel and help you feel full while you're breaking down fat cells. Glucagon also helps turn protein into sugar for energy. If your body is short of energy, it will pinch protein from your lean body. Eating adequate protein not only allows you to avoid muscle breakdown, but also fills you up. Converting protein to fuel takes time and costs the body energy, and the net energy you get from protein is less than from any other nutrient you eat. How do you trigger the release of the wonder-hormone glucagon? You eat protein.

Where protein is in chronically short supply, people develop a disease called marasmus, or wasting. If both protein and calories are lacking, the condition is called kwashiorkor. You may have seen photos of third-world children with this condition—emaciated, with bloated bellies.

In summary:

Lack of protein produces illness;

Lack of sugar produces health;

And vice versa.

The key to making protein work for you is to give your body a slow, steady supply of it. That means protein should be the core of every meal. Each meal should have a minimum of 15 grams of protein in it, and your distribution of it throughout the day should be as even as possible. This will maintain your blood sugar and keep you feeling full.

Anti-aging

You may know that one of the hallmarks of aging is loss of muscle and bone. A main component of both is protein. There is your first lesson in anti-aging. The other two are low sugar and moderate exercise. Long before you think of hormone injections, get your nutrition right— there's no substitute for that. If this sounds like the Food Tree, it's no coincidence.

To Be or Not to Be Vegetarian

Many of my patients are vegetarians. While I respect their views, I don't necessarily agree that we were created to live that way. If we don't eat meat, we may develop deficiencies of vitamin B12 and/or iron.

Picture the great beast hunt in ancestral times, with the group sharing the bounty. At a distance, one fellow says, "No, thank you, I'll just have a salad and a B12 supplement." Somehow, I just don't believe that's how it happened. Philosophically bad as it might be, I think we're omnivorous—we live at the top of the food chain, and always have.

Fat—Friend or Foe?

Fat is a much-misunderstood and maligned nutrient. I'm tempted to repeat what I said about protein: fat is your most important nutrient, and it needs to be the right kind.

Aside from energy storage, fat is an essential component of all our body cell walls. Fat provides insulation and carries vital fat-soluble hormones, enzymes, and vitamins around our bodies. It's also the basic building block of our now well-known super-hormones.

As a macronutrient, fat slows down the absorption of other nutrients and lowers the glycemic effect of carbohydrates. It's GI stabilizing, but not enough to offset the effect of the total load eaten. Chocolate and ice cream are relatively low GI, but they're high-fat items that are hard on the waistline because they pack a load of fat calories with enough sugar to store them quickly. We went through the low-fat/fat-free craze only to find our waistlines bigger than ever and our health failing.

Unlike sugar, fat doesn't rear the ugly head of insulin and your weight thermostat, and it's not addictive. We don't get fat eating fat. Who ever got fat drinking oil or eating butter or lard? Most of my patients who say they overeat on fat actually eat chips, French fries, pizza, crackers, and other carbohydrates that are laced with fat. Bad fat usually takes its toll by riding along with sugar. The carbohydrate part of these items raises insulin, facilitating storage of both the carbohydrates and the fat. If you burn all the energy you take in, whether it's from sugar or fat, your insulin will stay within the window and you won't gain weight. As you'll learn, your fat requirements are small, but the kind of fat you eat is crucial to good health.

Too much or the wrong fat becomes a *compound toxin* that adds insult to sugar-injury. Here's how it works: Animal fats eaten within the confines of normal weight are not considered harmful. Biochemically altered (trans) fats are damaging in any amount, because they weaken the cell walls. Over-consumption of omega 6 fatty acids puts you at risk for excessive linoleic acid syndrome, which by itself is strongly correlated with metabolic illnesses. You get omega 6 from the vegetable oils in deep-pan- and stir-fried food. Most fast food is loaded with all of the above and is very harmful. In summary, unless it's a good fat from the Food Tree, all fat has the potential to raise your blood lipids, clog your arteries, and put your body into an inflammatory state. Living in this culture, we all suffer a bit of linoleic acid syndrome (too much of it converts to omega 6. See page 49). It's relatively easy to stop eating bad fat because it isn't addictive. Most people can switch to olive oil, change the way they prepare food, go easy on the stir-fry, and add omega 3.

Note that linoleic acid syndrome creates the same downstream effect as is caused by too much sugar and insulin. Small world.

Saturated and Unsaturated Fats

Fats are divided into two main groups: saturated and unsaturated. The saturated fats found in animal products are solid at room temperature and are found in lard or butter, while unsaturated fats come from plant products and fish.

Partially Hydrogenated Trans Fats

We've learned to extract oil from plants on a large scale. These oils are unsaturated in their natural state. Some are chemically altered from this natural unsaturated state to be partially hydrogenated, as well as brought from their natural so-called cis configuration to the trans state. This raises their burning point and prolongs their shelf life, but it's very unhealthy for our bodies. These are the frying oils used commercially.

Partially hydrogenated trans fats are the hidden fats in fast food and processed foods, which damage you without your knowing it. Commercial baking fats and margarine used to be in this group, but due to toxicity, their use is declining.

Essential Fatty Acids

Ten percent of fatty acids in our bodies are polyunsaturated. Our body can't produce them, so they have to be ingested. They're called essential fatty acids (EFA). We know them in two biochemical varieties: omega 3 and omega 6. The basic ingredient of these is found in small quantities in almost all foods, especially fats, as a precursor named linoleic acid. Our bodies turn linoleic acid into either omega 3 or omega 6 depending on circumstances. Omega 6 fatty acids are found in most Vegetable oils (i.e. corn oil). Ready-made omega 3 oils are found in fish fat, almost-ready omega 3 in nuts (especially walnuts), flaxseed, canola, and wheat germ. We need a healthy balance of these two to keep our bodies' cells healthy. Omega 3 is crucial to brain-cell function. Along with cholesterol (yes, that's right), they encase the brain itself, something currently being explored by Alzheimer's researchers.

Furthermore, the omega 3 and 6 EFAs are the building blocks for what are known as our super-hormones. These hormones are like swift, strong extensions of insulin—and like insulin, they have a finger in every pie in the body. Together they decide how healthy you are!

Let's look at some of what they do. These super-hormones regulate:

1. the body's cell growth;
2. the flow of substances in and out of the cells;
3. oxygen transport;
4. nerve transmission;
5. inflammation;
6. allergic reactions;
7. blood clotting;
8. immune response; and
9. enzyme and hormone synthesis, especially steroids, which include the sex hormones—how's that for incentive to keep your insulin low?

So it's no exaggeration to say that the super-hormones run the show. Each time you eat, you decide whether all of these processes are going to run in your favor or work against you.

As long as omega 3 and omega 6 are in balance, we build good cell walls, produce good super-hormones, and stay healthy. If omega 6 takes over, we produce the wrong super-hormones, our bodies become inflamed, and we start showing ill health. As a culture, how are we doing at balancing our EFAs? We're woefully overweight and overdosed on omega 6 from high intake of processed vegetable oils and animal fat, and low intake of fish.

So how do you strike a balance? Omega 3 is the weakest link, and yields to the dominant omega 6 under the following circumstances: when you take in too much omega 6, when your glucagon is low (i.e., when your protein intake is low), and—most amazing—when your insulin is high, your super-hormone production is pushed toward overproduction of omega 6. And when is that? Your insulin is high by definition when you're overweight. We can reverse that ratio by lowering insulin, increasing glucagon, and ingesting omega 3 fatty acids while putting the brakes on our intake of linoleic/omega 6.

Unfortunately, our access to omega 3 is limited because our seafood supply is tainted with several toxins, including PCBs and mercury. The safest alternative is chemically purified omega 3 supplements. But above all, we need to lower insulin and keep our weight normal, or our enlarged fat cells will become factories spewing bad super-hormones regardless of what else we do.

You can now begin to see what I meant by saying that insulin is the master hormone of your health and weight. It shows up wherever there's important regulation of processes in your body. The type of fat you eat also makes or breaks your health.

So what about the saturated animal fats? It turns out that as long as you eat them within the confines of normal weight, and after you've eaten the necessary unsaturated fats to stay healthy, they might not be harmful to you.

Bringing Your Nutrition into Balance

Once your nutrition is in the kind of balance I've outlined so far, there's less room for things that harm you, because your body will feel full and shut off its weight thermostat. If your head still wants something after your body feels full, don't eat it—you'll gain weight. If you need a treat, and we all do, find one that works. Think about eating ice cream and chocolate in the way of the old saying about making love to a porcupine: very carefully!

Animal fats contain fatty acids we need, which means that lean meat and dairy are part of a well-rounded nutritional program. Manmade trans fatty acids are bad in any amount and should be avoided (margarine and other processed spreads, fats used in processed foods, baked goods).

So how much other fat do you really need, and what kind is good for you?

Let's look at olive oil. It's neither omega 3 nor omega 6, but omega 9, and neutral to your omega balance. The Mediterraneans have it right— most of their fat intake comes from fish and olives. In addition, they use a lot of vinegar and lemon juice which are biochemically defined as fatty acids. They slow down carbohydrate absorption, lowering GI.

Some 30 percent of your energy intake for the day should be from fat. Out of 2000 kcal, that would be about 600–700 kcal. This is equivalent to 3–5 tablespoons of olive oil, plus the fats you get from animal sources during a day's balanced eating.

If fish is mostly absent from your menu, you need to supplement with omega 3 oil capsules, taken as directed on the container labels.

All the fats we eat are transported in the bloodstream to their final destination. Some are used for energy, some end up being used by the liver, and some are used to maintain cells and other structures. Whatever we don't use, we store. If we overeat on fat, our bloodstream can literally turn creamy, completely clogging our blood vessels. We get the same damage from overeating on sugar, because the liver turns sugar into fat and sends it on its way to storage. The wrong kind of fat will damage the walls of the blood vessels as it passes through. Trans fat is incorporated into cell walls as faulty building blocks that will weaken the vessel.

So far we've talked about the so-called long fatty acids. Now to the medium-length fatty acids—the best known being palm and coconut oils. Totally saturated, they were thought to be very damaging until we studied the diet of Thai people, who use coconut oil as a frying staple. Thai people are thin and virtually free of heart disease. Medium-length fatty acids are now thought to be similar to saturated animal fat. Within the confines of normal body weight, saturated fats are not harmful, because they're burned as fuel before they can do harm.

Next are the short fatty acids. You know them as butyric acid (butter) and acetic acid—vinegar. Yes, vinegar is biochemically a fatty acid. I said that vinegar slows absorption of sugar through the GI-stabilizing property of all fatty acids, but this one doesn't put weight on you from fat calories! Butter also has nutrients, including carotenes, that are good for you. Again, in small doses butter is good for you. Some short fatty acids are made in your colon by bacteria that ferment fiber; they might help protect against colon cancer.

Cholesterol

Finally, there's cholesterol. Complicated and mysterious, cholesterol is a specialized member of the fat family. It's found exclusively in animal products because it's a necessary building block for healthy cell walls, including those of brain cells. It's also the basic building block for vitamin D, the steroid hormones (including sex hormones), and bile acids.

The reason it's targeted for endless scrutiny as the offender in heart disease is that cholesterol is what hits us in the eye when we look at plaques in damaged blood vessels. We know exactly how it got there. *Why* it got there is another matter.

Only about 15 percent of the cholesterol in your bloodstream is ingested through food. Your liver produces the rest of it—approximately 85 percent. You've been told that cholesterol comes from eating fat. Consult a biochemistry textbook and you'll see that the basic building unit of cholesterol is a different biochemical unit—an activated sugar molecule. Moreover, the rate-limiting step in cholesterol production is run by—you guessed it—our old friend insulin. Your liver turns sugar into fat and/or cholesterol, but only when your insulin is high.

Therefore we see that people who stop eating sugar lower their fat and cholesterol. We all know the model eater who can't lower cholesterol for love or money. Remember the normal distribution of human characteristics? Some people lack the enzymes to utilize lactose or other metabolites. Others may produce too much cholesterol, or may lack mechanisms to get rid of it. They may have a family history of high cholesterol, often combined with the early onset of heart disease. These are the patients who truly need lipid-lowering medications.

Is Cholesterol the Culprit?

There's a clear relationship between certain familial cholesterol patterns and heart disease. But as we've seen, when it comes to high cholesterol in general, the picture becomes more complex. There are studies that suggest that up to 80 percent of patients with coronary artery disease have the same cholesterol as those who don't have the disease.

Because we understand how the body metabolizes cholesterol, we can interrupt its metabolism in several places to lower production or excretion. The first step is to lower your insulin!

Is It Cholesterol or Sugar?

Remember the Johns Hopkins study of sugar as the cause of heart disease? It showed that in non-diabetics, blood sugar predicts heart disease better than any risk factor, including cholesterol. You can now understand this. If it's true that sugar raises insulin, that insulin turns on omega 6 production and pro-inflammatory hormones, causing a generalized inflammation in your blood vessels, and that this creates inflammatory cholesterol plaques in those same vessels, people with high blood-sugar levels should be at high risk, and vice versa. This has been demonstrated to be true.

People with high cholesterol are at increased risk for cardiovascular disease, but low cholesterol doesn't necessarily mean the same dramatic reduction of risk as we see with lowering sugar. Cholesterol is made from sugar. Meanwhile, we've become unhinged about fat and especially cholesterol, starting downstream in the chain of events, pummeling our cholesterol with statins to the tune of $10 billion per year, while we tolerate abnormal long-term blood sugars in diabetics and non-diabetics alike.

You've heard of the different types of cholesterol, and that lowering "bad" (LDL) cholesterol is crucial. As of this writing, scientists are conceding that lowered LDL cholesterol has not produced the anticipated decrease in heart disease. Unfortunately, cholesterol-lowering drugs lower "good" (HDL) cholesterol as well. And that might be a bad thing (see the American Heart Association's *Get With the Guidelines* program at www. americanheart.org). Scientists are now desperately lowering the norms for cholesterol again, still missing the obvious.

The fundamental issue remains addiction to refined sugars, compounded by bad fat. Sugar is the first link of the chain that leads to fat, cholesterol, and metabolic diseases, and should be our primary target in lowering cholesterol and reversing metabolic illnesses.

Our ancestors reportedly had an average cholesterol of 125. But no one talks about what their average blood sugar was. That would explain a lot of things, including their cholesterol.

You'll notice that the top of the Food Tree is small, shrinking with each piece of emerging information about sugar.

Removing not fat, but bad fat, is the other issue. Coronary heart disease was unknown to the Inuit when they lived on marine fat and protein. They had no carbs and negligible omega 6. I rest my case.

I also eat as though my life depended on my blood sugar. Oh, and I eat my protein, and cook my fish in olive oil.

I predict that within a short time, testing for long-term blood sugar will be routine in all patients. But testing doesn't heal anyone or anything. The Food Tree does.

So What About Taking a Pill?

An overview of the Food Tree will show you that it follows the principles of proper nutrition. *Learn to like what your body likes—food instead of sugar.* It's also about balancing nutrition and helping keep your blood sugar low and your body strong through activity. Instead of recognizing this, we're forever waiting for the silver bullet.

Ready for a leap of imagination? Here it is: A pill to remove sugar from our lives, thereby stopping metabolic illness right at the source. Preferably, it should remove the damaging types of fats as well. No side effects, reasonably priced, and self-directing—it would make us eat the right things at the right times and keep our bodies active. If only we had such a pill. The bad news is, no such pill is likely to be found. But the good news is, now that we know what we need to do, we have the opportunity to use our knowledge to do it.

Micronutrients

Micronutrients are nutrients you can't see: vitamins, trace minerals, and polyphenols. We may not be able to see them, but they're vital to every aspect of cell function. Without them, we develop deficiencies.

Vitamins and trace minerals are essential for running the body's metabolic processes. If we develop deficiencies, we'll eventually suffer distinct clinical syndromes associated with their lack. We've already discussed where they're found: Vitamins come from the vegetables and proteins included in the food groups. Trace minerals come from the ground; you access them by eating the things that absorb them— vegetables and fruits. Polyphenols are the little foot soldiers that keep your body processes running smoothly, keep your immune system strong, and protect your cells from undue wear and tear.

We have an interesting biochemical quirk about us: even when our metabolism runs normally, we produce molecules called free radicals that react with oxygen molecules and can damage our normal cells. This reaction is normally limited and we have natural defenses against it. If we suffer inflammation, exposure to toxins, or other stress, we produce more free radicals, and our natural defenses against them are overwhelmed.

Our nutrition should be geared toward neutralizing free radicals with foods that have antioxidant, anti-aging effects. And where do you find these anti-radicals? In the polyphenols that color fruits and vegetables— the more color, the more protection. How much is enough? Here's the good news: if we stop flooding our bodies with sugar, we make room for nutrition. If we eat a variety of foods, we'll get every micronutrient we need by association; we won't need to be experts on the latest and greatest flavonoid—we'll get them all!

Multivitamins Are an Insurance Policy

Because I want to cover all needs in weight loss, I give everyone a good multivitamin that includes trace minerals and flavonoids. See the list of the individual vitamins on page 131.

Have you noticed that no essential micronutrient comes from grains and sugar?
And neither does any essential macronutrient.

Nutrition and Good Health—Knowledge is Power

Completing the description of the various nutrients, it strikes me that I've used the word "vilified" about all the food groups. I think this is an expression of our ignorance, frustration, and feeling of utter powerlessness in our relationship with food. Rather than enlighten ourselves about it, allowing food to serve us as a positive element in life, we understand little about it and curse the darkness.

Do you love to eat? I hope you do—it's one of life's great pleasures. We should eat, drink, and be merry! Our relationship with food should be as powerful as our other relationships. Unfortunately, for some 70 percent of us the results of our eating are destructive. We're just not giving our bodies the building blocks they need. Rather than stones for bread, we're giving our bodies sugar for food.

The easiest way to gauge how things are going is by how well your wardrobe fits. Amazingly, we have no relationship with our bodies. We have no idea how they work or what they need to behave. Perhaps we don't want to know. You put your overweight, ailing body on a short-term diet to behave, and pummel it with metabolic garbage the rest of the time. When you punish your body, the results are never good.

Your body suffers in silence and compensates for this abuse for years, until it can't take any more, usually around middle age. You get a warning shot—a cardiac event, diabetes, or some other metabolic problem. If you survive, you're a lifestyle patient, and the torture of your poor, sick body continues.

Even more amazing, your weakened and abused body has incredible reserves and resilience to recover—if you give it a chance. What's more, it doesn't need much. You just need to stop feeding it garbage and start giving it the building blocks it needs. Food kills, but it also heals. Build a Food Tree for your body!

• Our misinformation about food is appalling. A friend of mine is taking medication for high cholesterol and is avoiding cheese. Meanwhile, he eats sugar freely. It's painful to watch him avoid a food that could yield protein and calcium and leave his insulin low, while raising his insulin with sugary "foods," thereby accelerating the transformation of sugar into fat and cholesterol.

Do I hear you questioning the dairy fat? Remember: eating these fats within the boundaries of normal weight is not harmful. There are also low-fat cheeses that are good options. In small doses even butter has fatty acids that are beneficial to us.

Another friend is very overweight and has heart problems. He's very proud of being a "good eater." I watched him eat a few vegetables and a sliver of steak for dinner, proudly announcing that he ate red meat sparingly, only to walk away hungry. He then ate a bowl of potato chips! Lean meat is a top-quality protein. This poor man ate a whopping dose of commercial fat along with enough potatoes to raise his insulin to store the stuff! Not to mention the salt (we'll get back to that). It was enough to make a nutritionist cry!

One patient, a nutritionist himself, told me he couldn't stop eating cake because if he did, the "hoarding principle" would appear later. Once we sorted out that his body cringed at the cake and hungered for real food, but that his head was stuck in the old addictive cycle, he smiled as the light came on instantly.

The Food Tree contains the right balance of macronutrients and micronutrients you need for good health. Now that you understand the basic principles of nutrition, it's time to build your Food Tree.

Here's a table of the contents of the Food Tree. We'll get more details on the exact amounts, plus a seven-day meal plan in chapter 5. Just as you know your own neighborhood, get to know your GI neighborhoods.

The Food Tree has four tiers, depicted on the next page, geared toward normalizing your blood sugar and keeping it there.

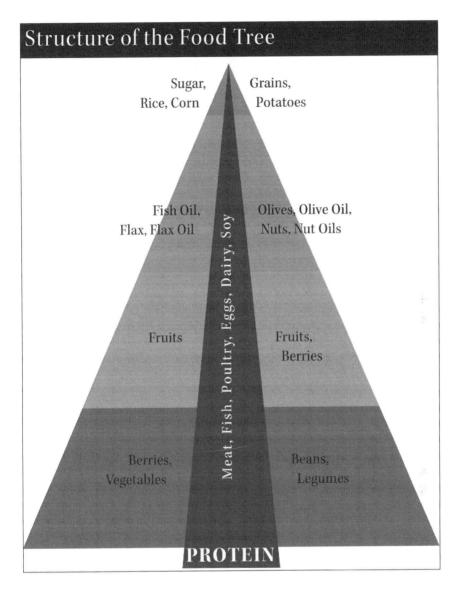

Structure of the Food Tree

Sugar, Rice, Corn

Grains, Potatoes

Fish Oil, Flax, Flax Oil

Olives, Olive Oil, Nuts, Nut Oils

Meat, Fish, Poultry, Eggs, Dairy, Soy

Fruits

Fruits, Berries

Berries, Vegetables

Beans, Legumes

PROTEIN

Components of the Food Tree

	GI	Composed of	Includes	Nutritional Value	Amount
Top Branches	50–100	High-GI Carbs	Pure sugars, sweets, milled grain, most breads, rice, potatoes	Quick energy only Toxic when overused.	Sparingly
Upper Branches	Help regulate GI	Unsaturated fats	Olive oil, fish, nuts, flaxseed/oil	Energy storage, support metabolic processes	See fat require-ments in chapter 4.
Middle Branches	40–50	Moderate-GI Carbs	Fruits, small amounts of pasta, whole and coarsely milled grain	Fuel, vitamins, minerals, polyphenols	Careful or they'll get in your way.
Low-lying Branches	0–40	Low-GI Carbs	Vegetables, legumes, berries, low-GI fruits	Fiber aids volume and digestion. Vitamins, minerals, and poly-phenols.	Consume 4–5 cups a day. Go easy on fruit in weight-loss mode.
Trunk	Helps regulate GI	Protein	Lean meats, fish, fowl, dairy products, eggs, soy	Building blocks for lean body and all protein-based cells.	See protein require-ments in chapters 3 and 4.

CHAPTER 5
Building Your Food Tree

N ow that you have a working understanding of your body's weight thermostats, together with the basic formula for regulating them, it's time to create your own Food Tree.

The Structure of the Food Tree

The Food Tree is based on the body's daily nutritional requirements: Lean protein and low to moderate glycemic-index carbs that keep our glucose-insulin (G-I) curve within the frames of the glucose-insulin (G-I) window. The right fats complete the balance to keep us healthy in weight loss and maintenance modes. When you eat these foods, your blood-sugar levels remain consistent throughout the day, you're not hungry, and you don't feel the ups and downs of a high-sugar diet. Eating this way will help put your body into balance with your health and weight.

If you're being treated for diabetes, kidney or liver disease, or any other medical condition, or if you take medications or have dietary restrictions, consult your doctor before you make any changes to your nutrition program. You might need to taper off medications and work closely with your doctor throughout.

Remember: You adjust your weight by controlling the slope and height of the G-I curve. The steeper and taller the curve, the more you store and gain weight. Any carbohydrate with enough sugar to put your G-I curve above the normal window increases your insulin levels and weight gain, skews your omega 3 vs. omega 6 fatty acid production toward inflammation, and weakens your health.

If your goal is to prevent or reverse diabetes, stay as close to the basic structure as you can.

We all should eat as though we're preventing diabetes, because we are!

Creating Your Food Tree

1. **Protein is the trunk of your Food Tree.** Trees need a solid

trunk. Once you put that in place, you can add the branches. Calculate your daily protein requirement, based on your needs. Remember: your protein requirements depend on your activity level (see formula on page 118). Divide your protein among your meals and snacks to keep the trunk of your Food Tree solid. Breakfast and each snack should contain a minimum of 15 grams of protein. Divide your remaining daily protein evenly between lunch and dinner.

2. The lower, thicker branches are the vegetables, legumes, and berries. Eat a minimum of four cups of vegetables a day—more is better. A serving of vegetables is one cup. Lettuce does not have much fiber; solid vegetables and legumes do. Mix them. If it's easier to find a salad for lunch, make sure your dinner includes fibrous vegetables. Berries are an excellent dessert or snack food. Your bulk comes from the lower branches of the tree. As you move up the tree, pick carefully to create a genuine Food Tree, not a garbage tree!

3. Next are the fruit branches. This category raises blood sugar in diabetics. If you're diabetic or trying to lose weight, 2–3 servings per day. Fruit has nutrients and fiber. If you're trying to lower your blood sugar, limiting this group will keep your GI low. Pasta is interesting in that GI is 40-50 or so, but that only takes 2 oz. to get to GI 13. Careful. Very coarse grains can dip under 50. Rice goes from high to low (wild rice 35).

4. The higher, smaller branches are your fats. You need 3–4 tablespoons of olive oil or other monounsaturated oils per day. While "smaller" here refers to physical amounts, fat is calorie dense and adds up quickly. It's important to spend your fat calories wisely; the wrong ones may be harmful. Exchanges for a tablespoon of olive oil: a tablespoon of butter, a tablespoon of mayonnaise, 10–15 nuts or olives depending on their size, a quarter to a half of an avocado. Nuts and olives are excellent healthy snacks that keep your GI low.

Note: For good health, I recommend that everyone take omega 3 oils, typically starting with fish and flaxseed oil in capsule form as directed on the container. If you eat a lot of fish, this is optional.

5. The smallest top branches are the sugars. This is the last thing you add to the top of your tree, as this is where you jolt your GI. You want to eat, cereal, bread, potatoes, rice, and corn as additives rather than as a food group. If you add this branch, make it short but sweet, so to speak. The best breakfast cereals are oatmeal or oat bran because of their relatively low GI and soluble fiber.

6. Build your tree around three meals and two snacks a day. This will keep your G-I curve even.

7. Plan and shop for your Food Tree on a weekly basis. Remember: You'll make up your tree from what's available. If you have the right foods around, chances are your tree will have the right proportions.

8. In weight-loss mode take in extra micronutrients. Take a good multivitamin daily, one that includes the most important trace elements and flavonoids, as well as calcium to protect your bones. The trace element chromium (also found in black pepper, brewer's yeast, mushrooms, prunes, raisins, nuts, and asparagus) is essential to weight loss and reduction of blood-sugar levels.

9. Drink adequate fluids to stay hydrated and to flush waste products. Two quarts a day of water is fine. Any non-caloric beverage, such as diet soda or other carbonated beverages, is okay if you prefer. If you're a coffee drinker, don't torture yourself thinking you have to quit to lose weight or to stay thin.

10. Salt (sodium) is clearly linked to high blood pressure. When you drink a high volume of water, you need some salt or you'll deplete your kidneys. Our western diet is high in salt, so you get enough through your food. Don't add extra salt.

11. Limit your alcohol consumption the way you limit your sugar intake. Remember that sugar and alcohol are the toxic cousins. If you enjoy alcoholic beverages, have one to two glasses of wine or one to two small drinks a day. Stay away from sweet mixers.

A Look at the Structure of a Typical Food Tree

Breakfast = 15 grams of protein; add allowed juice, fruit, coffee. Anything from your treat list if needed to feel full.

10:00 a.m. snack = 15 grams of protein; treats as needed.

Lunch = half of your remaining daily protein plus 2 cups of salad or vegetables/legumes.

3:00 p.m. = 15 grams of protein.

Dinner = your remaining protein for the day, plus 2 cups of vegetables/legumes/salad.

In addition: Eat 2–3 pieces of fruit at meals or as snacks. To get your daily amount of fat, use olive/canola/nut oils as dressing. Have appropriate treats if hungry at any time.

Cultivating a Balanced Tree

To cultivate a healthy, balanced tree, think in the following terms: If you're overeating on protein and not getting enough complex carbohydrates (fiber) and fat, you're left with a dry tree trunk. If you eat only the branch foods, your branches have nothing to attach to, and you won't have a tree, but a pile of branches on the ground. If you leave a branch out, there's a gap in your tree.

Your Food Tree in balance is the key at all times.

Note: If you don't have time for a 10:00 a.m. snack, you can add it to your breakfast or lunch, but the 3:00 p.m. snack is mandatory—always.

Losing Weight

The closer you stay to this basic design, the faster you'll lose weight. If you're hungry, you can eat more of anything on the basic tree. If you add sugar, you raise your insulin and slow your weight loss. Understanding this, make informed choices. The weight-loss version of your tree will result in a steady loss of about 1–2 pounds per week, without hunger or deprivation.

Note: How quickly you lose weight is based on the type of "loser" you are. Some people are genetically predisposed to lose more quickly (see chapter 3).

Maintaining Your Weight

In maintenance, your protein-trunk requirement drops to 1 gram per kilo of ideal body weight per day, plus allowances for special needs if you have them.

Think Mediterranean. Base your Food Tree on fresh ingredients, wonderful combinations, and easy preparation.

Increase your vegetables, fruits, and legumes first. Use legumes as a staple. Peas, beans, and squash make great side dishes. An occasional serving of bread, pasta, or rice is okay. Use wild rice (GI 35) if possible. Olives and nuts are terrific snacks. Dark chocolate has low GI; a small piece isn't the worst dessert you could have.

If your belt feels uncomfortably tight after a meal, your tree is becoming top-heavy and will collapse on you. If you're hungry after you've eaten a meal or a snack, your body is talking to you. Listen! It's telling you that it's missing food, not sugar. Your Food Tree's trunk is too weak (not enough protein), or your branches are too small (not enough bulk, i.e., vegetables). Eat more, but eat the things that keep your tree balanced and healthy!

Seven Days on the Food Tree

Make copies of the nutrition guide starting on page 121. Post it on your refrigerator and use it to create your weekly shopping list. You're shopping for your body. If you shop for your head, you might be wasting your calories on garbage and your body will suffer for it. Don't go shopping when you're hungry. Everything looks different if you do.

Here are some suggestions for each meal during a week on the Food Tree.

Breakfast choices (minimum 15 grams of protein)

Tomato or vegetable juice (V-8) if you're a juice lover.

Coffee, tea, or low-fat milk.

3 egg whites (one yolk is okay) or EggBeaters.® Scramble or make an omelet with any lean meat if you need to augment your protein, or with vegetables for bulk. Try Dr. Elvebakk's all-purpose/anytime frittata!

1 yogurt (add protein powder, cottage cheese or any other protein source to bring the protein up to 15).

Half a cup of cottage cheese, with fruit or berries on top if desired.

A serving (the size of a deck of cards) of lean breakfast meat or sausage/ham/smoked salmon.

Pancakes (see recipe).

A protein bar or drink.

10:00 a.m. snack choices (minimum 15 grams of protein)

Beef/salmon/tuna, or turkey jerky (watch the salt if you have high blood pressure).

Low-fat cheese sticks.

A glass of low-fat milk with the proteins to bring your count to 15 gm.

A protein bar or drink.

Lunch choices (half of your remaining protein)

Chef/Cobb/seafood salad (2 cups) with chicken/shrimp/meat/tofu/tuna; use your imagination.

Lean burger or veggie burger without bun, use lettuce/tomato.

If you prefer a hot lunch, any lean meat, soy product, or fish to fill your requirements, with 2 cups of veggies/salad.

3:00 p.m. snack choices (minimum 15 grams of protein)

Same as 10:00 a.m.

Dinner choices (half of your remaining protein)

Chicken/turkey/meat/fish, grilled, broiled, or barbecued.

Two cups of vegetables; steamed, stir-fried (misting pan with olive oil), boiled, seasoned.

Sugar-free Jell-O or chocolate pudding (top with cottage cheese, ricotta cheese, or yogurt for added flavor and a protein boost).

Yogurt, fruit, berries.

So you want a treat? No problem. On page 133 is a list of treats you can enjoy anytime in weight-loss or maintenance mode. It's designed to get you to think outside the box about treats—these will help you, not hurt you.

Sample Food Tree for Adult Male, 5'10" Tall

A man 5'10" tall who wants to lose weight needs 113 grams of protein a day (rounded off to 115 grams; see guidelines on page 118). If he exercises hard, he might need up to 10–15 percent more protein per day to feel full and repair muscle. This is the trunk of his Food Tree throughout the day.

He needs the following amounts of protein during the day: 15 grams at breakfast, 15 grams at 10:00 a.m., and 15 grams at 3:00 p.m., for a total of 45 grams. The remaining protein, 70 grams, should be divided equally between lunch and dinner.

His tree branches are a minimum of 4 servings (cups) of vegetables and 2–3 pieces of fruit. Legumes such as lentils, peas, or beans are filling and healthy. Five tablespoons of olive oil and omega 3 oils would round out his basic program.

Once he starts maintenance, his protein requirement drops to 75 grams per day (plus allowance for activity), and he needs to add more branch foods until he's full, starting low and working his way up the Food Tree. His use of sugar hinges on his activity level.

The Food Tree Gives You Diet Amnesty!

You can end your struggle with food right now. *You have Diet Amnesty!* Don't even think "diet." Think liking what your body likes. Think generosity toward your body. You're *giving* your body good health rather than starving it into weight loss. You're simply stopping the flow of garbage to make room for nutrients, and you're eating nutrients until you're full. Once your body gets the food it needs, it makes alphabet soup of it and puts it right where it belongs. In return, you get the body you want without struggling—not a bad deal!

Think like Lucy, a patient of mine, who remarked, "I can't believe it—I'm living normally and losing weight. Life is good!"

Remember, this plan is not "high protein" or "low" anything. It's not based on a fad. It's a *balanced* Food Tree, emphasizing the nutrients your body needs to be healthy.

Note: For food lists, portion sizes, nutritional information, and cooking suggestions consult the appendices.

The Food Tree—Your Body in Balance

Now that you've brought your Food Tree into balance, you'll feel physiologically full and you'll have great energy and peace around food. Instead of feeling helpless and confused, you'll feel informed and powerful in dealing with food and nutrition issues. Best of all, you'll end up at your best weight.

What if you're still left with hunger that isn't physiological; you simply crave something, though you might be full? This is when psychology enters the picture. Cravings are brought on by behaviors learned from your culture (well, maybe your genes play a part here)—we call them triggers.

Triggers leading to cravings are very common, and until you've learned to feel physiologically full, you might not even be sure if you're actually hungry or if you're just craving. Once you recognize cravings, what can you do to change them? We'll discuss that next.

CHAPTER 6
Tame Your Triggers

You now have all the information you need to create and use your Food Tree. If you're still unable to make it work, we need to look a little further.

We may respond to certain cues by eating even though we aren't hungry. These cues are called triggers, and our responses are called cravings. Many people think they have cravings until they eat properly and the desire to eat goes away. Their cravings simply resulted from poor nutrition. Some people can't even identify cues—they just crave, and most often sweets. If you're eating right (with the Food Tree, for example) and still want junk food, you're now dealing with cravings, which may run the gamut from bad habits to addiction, only this one isn't connected to food or the G-I curve. If you're one of the latter, there's news for you: Finnish researchers have identified a sweet-tooth gene.

You might have conditioned yourself to eat a sweet because it is 9 p.m. or because you're watching your favorite TV show, or you might be driven to eat at any time for no reason.

If you doubt that, meet Annette, a patient who came to my office extremely upset. She had dropped fifty pounds and was beginning to accept herself, but she felt that sugar cravings were disrupting her success, even to the point of waking up in the middle of the night, and threatening to derail her new life.

This adds an entirely other layer to our insulin-driven eating, and you can now begin to see why the sugar addict is always just a step away from the behavioral-addiction curve. You see, as well, that you can no more tell a sugar addict to eat a carrot than you can tell an alcoholic to binge on soda water. The person's awareness needs to be changed.

When we realize that sugar has this potential, we should stop discussing whether it's a toxin—no one overdoses on tofu at 3 a.m.!

Are you beginning to see something else? It was not like this thirty years ago. We carried the same genes, we're just drowning our genes in sugar. We have created this massive problem ourselves. Which of course means we can un-create it, but it will take some doing.

Do you have triggers? If they run like tapes, they most likely end with you eating sugar.

The key is to recognize the tapes when they come on. This awareness may give you a chance to stop and change the end result by substituting another activity for eating. Achieving this level of self-awareness can take a little time. It requires a bit of introspection, to see where you may be prone to one or more of the ten problem eating patterns described below. This interesting exploration can be liberating. In fact, what you find out may interconnect with other areas of your life. When you get to the bottom of why you overeat, you could come away physically and emotionally lighter for your efforts. Shifting your behavior can bring you all kinds of interesting results.

On the other hand, hard-core sugar addicts like Annette need to find a way to stop bathing their genes in sugar. It takes support. I showed Annette all the coping techniques and connected her with a group of individuals who shared her problem. She also sought additional counseling, and is doing very well.

Identify Your Eating Triggers and Change Your Rewards/Treats

The best way to uncover your eating patterns is to follow the Food Tree. This way, you'll know your cravings aren't due to bodily hunger.

When you want to eat, simply ask yourself: "Am I actually hungry, or am I trying to fix something else? What am I trying to fix?" ("What's on my tape?") The following questions may help you answer.

Do you find that you make poor eating decisions when you're involved in specific social activities?

Do you end up eating too much or the wrong things when you're with certain people?

Are you a closet eater? Do you eat when no one is looking?

Which emotions induce you to eat?

To help you further identify your patterns, look over the following descriptions of ten problem eaters. Do any of these describe you? Do you identify with more than one? If so, try the suggested antidotes.

TEN PROBLEM EATERS

1. The Sugar Addict

The sugar addict is the genuine article. Like Annette, you're battling a real addiction. The pattern is classic: One cookie leads to a donut, then a candy bar, and then perhaps another cookie—or five. You find it difficult to have only one serving of rice or pasta. If someone puts a basket of bread in front of you, you devour it. You never seem to be satiated until you're totally sugar-loaded. You trigger on very small amounts of sugar in any form. The extreme sugar addict even triggers on fruit!

Antidotes for the Sugar Addict

Keep up your protein and find substitutes for sugar. Find an alternate food that will trigger your body into thinking it has had its sugar fix. It may take a little detective work to discover the craving-arresting food that works best for you, but sooner or later you'll hit on it. For example, one of my patients is a real chocoholic. We've been able to curb this craving by replacing her chocolate candy with a delicious, low-calorie, chocolate-flavored protein shake. Chocolate-covered protein bars are also available. Sugar-free Jell-O and other puddings will do as well.

Develop limitations. Do not keep sugar in the house. One of my patients swears by the scheduled treat—one scoop of ice cream twice a week. She eats it while out, if possible. This keeps her from feeling deprived. Say your affirmation # 2 (see chapter 7) "Sugar is toxic waste, I don't like it." Say it because the first part is true. Keep on saying it because the second part will ring truer the longer you say it.

Find your soul mates. It's very important for you to find others who understand how you feel. Your condition is real, and others who have it will recognize it. Support groups can be a tremendous asset and help you find solutions you hadn't thought about.

Most important, change your tape. If you can recognize when the tape starts running, you have a chance to stop it using any of the techniques above or by developing something that works for you. You might benefit from counseling.

2. The Food Lover

If you're a chronic food lover, you eat too much simply because you love the taste of food. Instead of eating to live, you live to eat. You get pleasure from various flavors and textures. There's nothing wrong with enjoying food, of course. It's one of life's great delights, and everyone deserves to take pleasure in it. If you go overboard, however, you need to implement strategies to modify the tendency.

Antidotes for the Food Lover

Sit down. Don't eat standing up or walking around—enjoy your meal at a table. When you eat on the run, it doesn't feel like you've eaten and it doesn't fill you up the way a sit-down meal does. It simply doesn't register as well with your satiety mechanisms.

Use smaller plates. Smaller plates give the appearance of more food. You don't need fourteen spoonfuls of anything to taste and enjoy it. I often remind my patients that the first spoonful tastes better than the fourteenth one. Savor the flavor rather than the amount. And savor the moment. Another reason why smaller plates are better is based on cultural norms. Some people belong to the "Clean Plate Club." They were raised to believe that when they leave food on their plate, they're wasting it—a true sin in some cultures. If you feel this way, use a smaller plate. It will automatically do something you might need to do: reduce your portion sizes.

Eat slowly and enjoy. If you love food beyond measure, learn how to enjoy food *in* measure. You'll find that an eight-ounce steak, eaten slowly during a nice meal, can bring as much pleasure as a sixteen-ounce steak gobbled voraciously.

Replace harmful food with healthy food. If you do eat that eight-ounce steak, make sure it's a lean cut instead of a fatty one. By doing so, you can reduce the amount of calories you eat by as much as 50 percent. This strategy works well because it doesn't leave you feeling deprived. You're simply substituting damaging food with a desirable, healthy selection. One of my former patients loved ice cream. I helped him to substitute yogurt, which he chilled to nearly frozen before eating. It's now his favorite dessert, yielding honest-to-goodness nutrition and fullness. One of my maintenance patients has replaced potato chips and corn chips with fat-free cheese strings and fat-free beef jerky, both of which satisfy his desire for something savory while coming close to being pure protein. Ted, another patient, struggled for a long time, and then one day came in and exclaimed, "I get it—I don't need the heavy chocolate to enjoy dessert. Now that I'm off sugar, I can appreciate the complexity and intensity of an orange. I love it!"

Replace eating with other activities. Do the things you love: Read a book. Rent a video. Call or visit a friend. Work on those new hobbies. As the old saying goes, "Idle hands do the devil's work."

3. The Environmental Cues Eater

A French proverb states, "A good meal ought to begin with hunger." All too often, however, eating begins with an environmental stimulus. For example, you see a sign advertising 31 flavors of ice cream and you pull over, contemplating the various choices. Or you begin to munch on a bag of potato chips, only to realize that you saw a commercial for chips moments earlier. You are an environmental-cues eater.

Environmental food cues can also come to you through your nose. How many times have you entered a movie theater not thinking about food until the smell of popcorn hit you? And why do you think bakeries vent their ovens over the front door? They want to lure you into impulse eating. Sometimes the very sight of food can prompt you to eat. You may mindlessly grab a candy bar at a checkout stand just because it's there, or you may elect to have a croissant simply because you saw it displayed in a pastry shop window. The old joke: "I'm on the seafood diet; when I see food I eat it" hits a little too close to home for you.

Antidotes for the Environmental-cues Eater

Recognize knee-jerk reactions. When you suddenly feel the need to eat, ask yourself these trigger questions: "Am I actually hungry, or is something else making me want to eat? What else might be making me crave food right now?" Try to identify what in your environment could have triggered your craving. If you can pinpoint something, tell yourself, "I won't let that stupid advertisement or marketing ploy tell me what or when I should eat!" Channel your so-called hunger into appropriate indignation.

Eat something healthier. When you're besieged with a craving initiated by something around you, ask yourself, "If my body really needs food right now, is this particular item what the *lean me* requires?" Reflect on the nutritional value of the cued item. If it's not something that will help you keep your setpoint turned to low, eat something that will instead.

Identify hunger accurately. As an environmental-cues eater, you've actually become deaf to the real hunger signals your body sends you. You may be chronically undernourished. If your nutrition is good and you're eating because "it's there," then it's time to recognize when you're truly hungry and train yourself to wait for that signal before eating. Sometimes, you'll discover that you've been listening to the wrong cue. Some patients, for instance, read the tiredness they feel after eating a carbohydrate-dense meal as a sign that they haven't eaten enough. In fact, just the opposite is true. Eventually, they come to realize that the sluggishness that follows overfeeding is different from the fatigue engendered by actually needing more food.

4. The Boredom Eater

When you're bored, you try to find ways to stimulate your mind and body. Thin people turn to reading, letter writing, walks, and other kinds of activities. Overweight individuals turn to food.

Antidotes for the Boredom Eater

Recognize the pattern. Sometimes, merely becoming aware that you eat when you're bored is enough to halt the practice. Talk to yourself about what you're doing. Tell yourself, "I was going to eat those leftovers because I'm restless. I'm going to call my sister instead." These internal dialogues can make eating a decision, not a reaction.

Develop hobbies and interests. The best vaccine for boredom eating is having lots of activities that you enjoy. Busy people tend to be too involved in life to dwell on food. I teach my patients to respond to boredom with exercise. Go for a walk, sweep out the basement and wash the car instead of taking it to the car wash. Thus you replace a damaging action with one that supports your new lifestyle and your lower body-weight setpoint.

Avoid boredom noshing at parties. It's possible to be surrounded by a sea of people at a party or public event, yet still feel bored. Don't fall victim to this kind of eating trap. The first time I attended a Super Bowl party, for example, even the handsome men sitting around the TV couldn't hold my attention through all the talk about touchdowns, field goals, and quarterbacks. I started munching on the lean, herbed tri-tip steak I'd brought for the potluck. As my boredom grew, I found myself attacking the coleslaw, which was made with full-fat mayonnaise.

After gazing vacuously at the TV screen some more, I returned to the table for chips and dip. Soon I was moving to the bucket of deep-fried chicken. I topped it off with a brownie I didn't really want. By that time, I was feeling sluggish, bloated, and hypocritical. The moral: either avoid gatherings where you know you'll be bored, or learn to recognize when you're bored at a party and sip water or juice instead of turning to the snack table.

5. The Stress Eater

Do you use food as a tranquilizer, reaching for a snack when workplace pressures or other stresses mount? Stress eating is, to use an expression from the old country, "like peeing in your pants on a cold winter day." It may provide instant warmth and comfort, but you'll soon regret it!

Antidotes for the Stress Eater

Ask yourself, "Am I really hungry?" As with the other types of reactive eating that we've already examined, eat mindfully by checking in with yourself. If you're truly hungry, ask yourself whether the item you're about to eat will feed your *lean body* or serve as fertilizer for your fat cells. If your hunger is really just a veiled form of anxiety, remind yourself that overeating would only *add* to your stress.

Enjoy soothing or energizing foods. Try a cup of green tea! It's a powerhouse of antioxidants and is very soothing to frayed nerves. And learn to love fruit, if you don't already. It's full of energy, plus fiber, and is one of nature's best sources of sugar. Did you remember to drink your water?

Find other ways to relieve your stress. Do breathing exercises, take a walk, or go to the gym. Learn some form of meditation practice. Have a coffee date with a friend to talk things over, or work with a counselor. If you have trouble dealing with the stress in your life, take a course in stress management. Employers, community colleges, and learning exchanges often teach stress-management skills.

Take control of the moment. I worked with Bob, a businessman who had been a stress eater all his life. Through self-study, he realized that he chronically reached for food when things in his work or personal life were running amok. I helped him to reframe his stress-related cravings as opportunities to be in control. Now, when Bob finds himself reaching for a candy bar or about to order too much at a restaurant, he stops and tells himself, "The only thing I can control right now is my eating, and by God, I will! I refuse to let my eating get out of control, too." Bob is no longer a stress eater.

6. The Loneliness Eater

If you're this kind of person, you eat for love, in a sense. During the day, your work routine may keep you from dwelling on your limited social life, but when you're alone, especially at night or on weekends, you search for solace in eating.

Antidotes for the Loneliness Eater

Get up and out. If you find yourself reaching for food to stave off solitude, walk or drive to the nearest cafe and enjoy a cup of coffee or tea. Read a book at the local library instead of in your living room. Browse a bookstore or your favorite shop, or explore a new town center that you've always driven past. Listen to music at a local venue. Just being around other people can banish those feelings of loneliness. You might even make a new friend. Better yet, put yourself in a situation in which meeting others is expected. Join a club or a social group—a book club, for instance. Treat your feelings of social isolation with a dose of other people, not food.

Seek the love you need. Once you begin to lose weight, chances are you'll feel more deserving of friendship and romance. This is what happened with my patient Martha. She lost twenty pounds, joined a dance club, and was soon waltzing steadily with a wonderful gentleman. She even brought him to meet me! Take advantage of your well-earned momentum by seeking out social situations and developing the relationships you need and deserve. Your improved appearance will help, but more significant will be your enhanced self-esteem and confidence. Self-assurance is very sexy! By developing interpersonal connections, you'll create a positive spiral in your life: the more weight you lose, the more you'll seek out others' company, and the less you'll find yourself eating out of loneliness.

Work with a counselor on relationship issues. You might need a little extra help from a professional to address interpersonal issues that could be preventing you from creating healthy relationships. My patient, Sasha, lost forty pounds, transforming herself from a rather corpulent matron to a svelte woman. Although she had overcome most of her poor eating habits, Sasha still had a problem with loneliness eating at night. Through counseling, she realized that she was still mourning her father's death. This grief would surface in the quiet evening hours, leading her to overeat. She worked successfully with a counselor to confront her feelings of loss, and has maintained her new body ever since.

7. The Depression Eater

If you turn to food when you're feeling down, you're probably a depression eater. Loneliness and depression eating often go together, because dissatisfaction with one's social life is among the things that can lead to depression. You may rely on specific comfort foods when you're feeling low, especially if your mother gave them to you to lift your mood when you were a child. If so, you learned at a very early age to use food to medicate yourself against negative feelings.

Antidotes for the Depression Eater

Reach for a pen, not a pizza. When you feel low, don't automatically head for the refrigerator. Instead, find a quiet place to reflect upon what you're feeling, and why. Think of what you need to do to address the cause of your depression. Write these thoughts down in a journal. Share them with a friend.

Get physical. Exercise has been proven to elevate mood. Regular walking or jogging helps increase your endorphins, your body's feel-good chemicals. A long walk may be all you need to put yourself on the better side of things. Sometimes a shower or a hot bubble bath can lift your spirits as well. Some authorities believe that heat increases serotonin levels in the brain, which heightens feelings of well-being.

Treat yourself to a pleasurable activity. Kick back and read your favorite magazine while sipping herbal tea. Listen to music you love. Browse the Internet. Watch an entertaining film. Indulge yourself with non-edible pleasures.

Find a good mental-health professional. As with loneliness eating, it can be important to work with a counselor to help you identify and come to grips with the life experiences that have led to your present depression. Sometimes quiet reflection isn't enough. A few of my patients feel they have issues that make it useful to supplement their weight-control programs with regular sessions with a psychotherapist.

8. The Reward Eater

You just got a promotion, and boy, are you happy. Your spouse says, "Let's celebrate!" Soon you hit the all-you-can-eat buffet, stuffing yourself with artery-clogging foods and sweets. If this sounds familiar, you're the type of person who rewards success with what amounts to a physical assault on your body. Again, this pattern may have started in childhood. Did your parents give you a cookie when you earned an "A" on a test? Did your coach take the team out for burgers if you won a Little League game? Did your Sunday-school teacher reward attendance by providing confections to those who came to class? These were meant as loving gestures, but now you need to love yourself enough to stop rewarding your success with food.

Antidotes for the Reward Eater

Find alternative rewards. To celebrate that promotion, for example, you and your partner can go for a scenic drive, stopping for a shrimp cocktail or creative salad when you're hungry. Or the two of you can see a movie or go shop for something you've always wanted and can now afford.

There's nothing dreary about eating well. Live high on the hog— just make it Canadian bacon!

9. The Broken-thermostat Eater

I've told you about the weight thermostats available to you. In some individuals they're simply weak or absent. I've seen this in a few patients, whom I call broken-thermostat eaters. Their self-regulating thermostats are always switched to the on position. They simply don't recognize the feeling of fullness, no matter how much they eat. They consume whatever food is present and leave the table only because others do. Today, medical science doesn't recognize this syndrome because we don't have biochemical markers to test for it. These are the people who really benefit from appetite-suppressant medication, because it resets their thermostats.

Antidotes for the Broken-thermostat Eater

Work with a physician. Because the biochemical functioning of the brain's appetite centers is not yet completely understood, there's no simple test to diagnose whether your thermostat is broken. An experienced weight-control physician, however, should be able to spot the problem by identifying certain patterns in your eating. The answer for you may be a treatment combining weight-control drugs and careful nutritional training.

Linda came to my program with a food history that revealed that her internal thermostat was indeed not working well. Good nutrition didn't change this. Although I don't normally advocate drugs, I felt justified in putting Linda on appetite suppressants while teaching her all about her biochemistry and proper nutrition. She returned in tears, thanking me for helping her experience what it means to leave the table full. In the absence of a well-functioning thermostat, you might need to use weight-control drugs, along with careful monitoring of your total caloric and nutrient intake, even to the point of keeping a food log every day and eating "by appointment only."

10. The Obsessive-Compulsive Eater

Are you obsessive-compulsive in other areas of your life? Do you sometimes have an overwhelming urge to eat? Do you often realize while eating that you're not hungry, and hate yourself for what you're doing? Do you binge eat? If you engage in any of these behaviors, you may be an obsessive-compulsive eater. The origins of obsessive-compulsive disorder, in general, are often hidden from view. Difficult to see, they can be even more difficult to change.

Antidotes for the Obsessive-Compulsive Eater

Start by gaining insight. Look at other areas of your life. Are you hard on yourself in general? Can you let things go, or do you get stuck?

Get mental health counseling. Obsessive-compulsive overeating may require treatment on several levels. If you want to move further toward comprehensive healing from this disorder, begin by working jointly with a psychologist, who can counsel you, and a psychiatrist, who can coordinate drug-treatment solutions. A counselor should help you identify what kinds of situations trigger your eating behavior and how the pattern came to be established . Psychiatric drugs may be useful in helping control anxiety and compulsive urges.

Some Tips for the Smoker

If you're a nonsmoker, you can skip this section. Current and former smokers often have difficulty managing their weight. This is true for several reasons. First, tobacco is a stimulant that increases your metabolic rate. If you quit smoking, you'll need to compensate for this decrease in your metabolism, which you can do by reducing your caloric intake, increasing your activity level, or both. Initially, eating less can seem difficult because the appetite-suppressing action of the nicotine will be gone. If you find yourself craving food more after you quit smoking, you'll need to find less-damaging ways to satisfy your urges. Reach for a vegetable snack or non-caloric beverage instead of potato chips or soda, for example.

Keep in mind that smoking is also a hobby. It has given you something to do with your hands and your mouth. Find alternative activities to keep them busy. For your hands, consider buying a hard rubber stress ball or take up doodling. For your mouth, invest in sugar-free mints or gum.

For many individuals smoking provides a basis for social bonding. Find healthier circles to interact with, such as a support group for people who wish to quit. It can be quite challenging to keep your focus on weight control when you're coping with smoking cessation. Don't try to transform yourself from an overweight smoker into a thin nonsmoker all at once. Make these changes gradually. For instance, as you work toward becoming an ex-smoker, set the modest goal of maintaining your current weight during the cessation process. Once you've overcome your addiction to tobacco, then move on to weight control.

I've found that individuals who are or have been smokers often have to work harder at weight control. A recent review of more than fifty papers on the nutritional habits of smokers indicates why this is so.

Jean Dallongeville and colleagues reported in their 1998 review, published in *The Journal of Nutrition*, that smokers tend to consume more calories, more total fat, more of the worst types of fat, less fiber, and less of several types of vitamins than their nonsmoking counterparts. Clearly, smoking is associated with a particularly unhealthy eating pattern that requires great effort to reform. At the same time, when patients tell me that they've conquered smoking, I know they have the capacity to make dramatic changes in their nutritional lives!

Share Your Reflections

Identifying and putting a lock on your eating triggers can be greatly aided by the support of both a counselor and a weight-control doctor. Qualified medical guides can help direct you in your own self-study by posing questions, providing diagnostic exercises, and giving suggestions. Bear in mind that this process takes time.

You may also benefit from the next chapter, which shows you the very interesting process of consciously working with mind technologies to help transform your mental energy and your life.

CHAPTER 7
Use the Power of Your Mind

Many of my patients who want to start eating according to the Food Tree guidelines find they need an extra boost to change a lifetime of bad habits or addiction. Is this your situation? If so, a powerful source of support is always there to help you. You can find it within yourself—it's the power of your mind.

Do you think you're overweight because you lack willpower or discipline? You now understand that that's just not true, and that kind of thinking lands you in a ditch. Willpower is not real power, because it's based on the notion that you're a struggling victim and must sacrifice to lose weight. When you make the choice to live a healthy life, you become a very powerful person. When you live by your convictions, the only thing you sacrifice is the victim mentality. Let it go—it wasn't serving you anyway.

Real power lies in understanding how to change what doesn't work into something that does, getting the results you want, and declaring yourself a winner. To gain real power, you must understand where power comes from and how you can use it to free yourself from the chains of the culturally implanted messages that have addicted and victimized you.

Your thoughts shape your life. They also shape your brain. This startling discovery has prompted medicine to start considering how our thoughts influence our bodies. This integration shapes everything in your life, including your weight and your health. Doctors call this holistic approach to health *integrative medicine*. It's nothing new—integrative medicine has existed for centuries, but during the past few years we got so preoccupied with lab results and X-rays that we forgot this mind/body connection.

Research is beginning to show that power in our lives comes from powerful thoughts. They become a mental energy field that creates our reality. The more focus we give these thoughts, the more power we have. When the mind and body work together, we create a very strong focus in any area of life. As insulin is the master regulator of our metabolism, our mind is the mainframe—the master control for everything that happens in our lives, including our ability to manage weight.

Our environment influences the way our thoughts are programmed. Negative thoughts or voices from as far back as our childhood produce limitations in what we think we're capable of. We listen to these thoughts when we fail at something and don't understand why. The real reason we failed was not, of course, that we couldn't do what we attempted, but that we didn't have the information and confidence to make it work. We have to get rid of these thoughts or voices, because they waste our mental energy and prevent our getting what we want.

With respect to your weight and health, just think of the little voices in your head that keep you from treating your body right. "I can't give up sugar." "It's hard to lose weight." Those are the voices of a powerless, addicted person. Even if we know what we need to do, we still might not be able to do it because we have no mental power in this area of our lives.

How much power do you have in your life? Look at what you have. It reflects your power. Are you spending your life in scattered energy—worse, in negative energy? The mental energy we use when we chat with someone at a party is pleasantly scattered and different from the power we call on when we concentrate to learn something.

Our thoughts are actually powerful enough to produce measurable changes in blood pressure and brain chemistry, and even change the appearance of a brain scan. If you have problems with your weight, look at your thoughts around weight: they may be mis-programmed. You're addicted, resigned, and passive—wasting all the mental energy available to you by accepting defeat. "I'm just too weak, lazy, old" etc. Don't let your thoughts create a world of distorted reality and mistaken identity wherein you are a willing victim.

Our subconscious controls our brain's programming automatically and follows these rules:

The Law of Attraction

I receive whatever I focus my energy on.

This is age-old wisdom. Most cultures have their version of it, expressed as something like "Be careful what you wish for, you might just get it!" What it really says is that you don't necessarily get what's best for you, but what you're calling toward you.

We may not be consciously wishing that bad things would happen to us—but by focusing our energy on a negative result, we might as well be bringing it into existence.

If you say you want to eat healthily, but spend your energy thinking about French fries, guess what will come to you? It's not about what you say, but where your energy really flows. Replaying our old mental programs keep us powerless.

Like other energies, mental energy can be positive, negative, focused, or scattered

Joy and gratitude are uplifting, positive thoughts. Concentrate on the word "joy" for a minute and you'll start smiling—that is positive energy! Stress, anger, and fear are negatives; try them and see for yourself. The harder you concentrate on joy, the better you feel, and vice versa.

Now think of the energy of sunlight, pleasantly scattered over the earth to light it up. But focus it into a laser beam and it becomes a whole other force, capable of incinerating matter. So it is with your thoughts. The life-altering power available to you if you learn to channel your mental energy is amazing. On the other hand, if you keep your energy puttering on "idle," you'll miss out on things you wanted but couldn't realize because you never learned to use your own mental power.

You can only focus your mental energy on one thing at a time

When your energy is caught up in fighting something negative, you have no energy to spend on positive things, and the outcome is always negative.

If you're resentful that some people's metabolisms differ from yours, and they can eat more and be thin, you have no energy left to create a plan for yourself to get what you want. Instead, you get stuck in the "life's not fair" mode, one of the most dangerous (i.e., negative) places to be. If you don't accept that we're all different, you'll have a lot of grudges to carry!

The Law of Reciprocation of Energy

I get back the same energy I send out.

You've heard people say that mood is one of the most contagious conditions around, and you've heard the expression "vibes." That's nothing more than others picking up on the thought energy you send out. Have you ever met a real con artist? The part you probably remember is the vibe this person gave off. The con artist's greatest skill is the ability to use his energy to make people feel dangerously good about themselves.

Conversely, think about your vibes the next time you're in a bad mood. You're simply broadcasting negative energy, which spreads like wildfire and eventually comes back at you with the same force you put behind it.

How Do We Apply These Rules to Eating?

What happens when you spend your energy obsessing about a slice of cake, thinking about it negatively to try to deny yourself what you want? You end up eating a slice of cake, because that's where you directed your energy, leaving you none to spend on something positive, something good for you, like a piece of fruit or cheese.

What if you decide the slice of cake is positive, you eat it, and then later feel guilty and negative about it? What's happened is that, in a short time, you've changed the way you think about a thing from positive to negative, and the thing suddenly changed! The final scenario is, you decide that cake is a negative, but this time you waste no time on it and send your energy toward a piece of fruit instead. When you direct your energy to that fruit, you've got no energy left to spend on cake, and you'll love your fruit and not miss the cake at all.

You've just discovered the final principle we'll use.

When You View Something Differently, It Changes

The cake is still cake, but your energy around it has changed, and cake no longer gets in the way of what you want, because you're not spending energy on it. In reality, you haven't given up anything; you've simply turned your attention to the things that make your life more positive. In other words, when you change the way you look at cake, cake loses its power over you.

When we're positive and focused, we have the power to bring into our lives what we want. When we dissipate our energy—or worse, waste it on negative thoughts—we're stopped in our tracks.

In this chapter, you've learned how to direct your energy from negative to positive to take power in your life. But how do we actually use this energy to become powerful? How do we turn our unproductive behavior into behavior that works?

Real power comes to your life if you take control. That's when you actively design and carry out your own changes, rather than waiting for something to happen.

You can change your reality to make anything happen by changing your thoughts.

This is known as mental reprogramming. That means deliberately changing your energy around something—in this case nutrition and weight. Since our destructive behavior happens on a subconscious level, the challenge requires not only laying down productive new circuits, but also erasing the old, unproductive ones.

Mind Technologies Can Change Your Reality

There are various techniques for reprogramming our minds: meditation, hypnosis, counseling, and analysis. They all aim to access the subconscious to allow true change to occur. The goal is to free your mind, allowing you to change your thoughts in an area of your life, so you can achieve what you want. Most of these methods are time-consuming and require a serious long-term commitment. Because of this, they're out of reach for many people. But there's a faster way to reprogram your inner computer and change those inner messages.

Affirmations Work—Big-time

You might be familiar with mantras or affirmations. They're no new invention. Eastern cultures have worked with them for millennia. Mantras are reprogramming "bytes" in the form of positive statements that are repeated daily to help us change our flow of energy. They're very powerful techniques, because they're easy to do and can be incorporated into most lifestyles. Best of all, they work.

We already know the power of mantras in what the advertising industry calls "messaging." They've shaped us for years, including our weight. Remember "You deserve a break today?"

Unfortunately, we aren't using the principle of messaging to our own advantage. We tend to snicker and call it "new-age stuff." Our loss. There's nothing "new age" about 5,000 years of experience.

A concept or product is associated with a positive saying—it's simple, to the point, and is repeated till it sticks. These are nothing more than mantras thrown at us until we act on them. I'd bet you think of "The Energizer" as "good" when you buy batteries! And you surely know who tells you they make the tastiest pizza in your town. So you see, you're already using mantras—except you're on the wrong end of them!

Do you see how the mantras that inundate and run you have power over you?

Then you also see how you could turn the tables. You can create your own personal message and use the power of messaging to get what you want, not what they want you to want.

When done right, mantras don't bring us what we want because we want it. Rather, they align our energy with our goals. They allow a state of concentration in a short time that gives us access to our subconscious and allows us to see how much power we have. They are calls to action that we send to our inner core to reprogram the computer. Wishing for something you want is not a mantra. But focusing your energy and visualizing yourself getting there will help you unleash the creative energy you need to get there. In other words, mantras mobilize your resources to make things happen. They also allow you to listen to the real power struggle in your mind that, though hidden from you, determines the outcome.

You've heard that positive energy works. Positive energy itself is a mantra. Optimism keeps you creative and looking for solutions, as opposed to fear, which paralyzes you and stops your creative flow. Done right, mantras speed up your growth—if you do whatever else it takes to get you there.

So, how do we create an effective mantra and use it? The first premise is that our goal can't be outlandish and unrealistic. We have to stake our energy on a reachable goal. I've already shown you that losing weight is a very attainable goal, on a purely scientific basis. Now you need to focus the power of your mind on implementing what you want.

Remember: Breathing a wish to the wind as we rush off in the morning doesn't open any doors to change. Your mantra needs to reach inward.

How to Practice Your Mantra

You have to take time out and feel focused and calm. You then compose a declaration of your goal in the present tense, starting with: I, (your name), am becoming/am doing, etc. Then you state your plan, how you're going to do this.

For instance: "I, Ann, am becoming so thin because I give my muscles protein."

That's the first mantra I teach my patients. It's very specific, pinpoints a goal, and states a workable plan to get there. You can think it or say it aloud.

You now give yourself time to hear the little voices in your brain— these are your software errors. They might say, "But you know you failed before, this won't work, you can't live without eating pizza," etc. What do you do now? You repeat your mantra, a little louder, directed at the little voices. You listen again, you repeat, ever louder. You might write it down. You repeat until it starts dominating your internal conversation and the negative voices fade away. You're slowly writing over an old slate, full of messages that don't work for you, with messages that do. When the positive message is the only one left, your energy will be centered on it, and it will change your energy.

Rather than short-order miracles, your mantras are tools for you to grow into a person who can make your mantras come true. Practice them regularly and you can reprogram yourself as well as any TV commercial. You'll be amazed at your progress as your new, more positive program helps you accomplish what you want.

I've had extraordinary success in changing people's eating habits by messaging information to them this way.

If you're a scientist, call your messaging commercial breaks. From research, you already know that they work. If you're a spiritual person, I submit to you that you weren't created to be fat. You became fat because your mind lost touch with your body. Your body is suffering, and you're in disharmony between your body and mind. To restore harmony, you need to get your mind to listen to your body. To that end, eating is a spiritual issue. It's about bringing harmony into your life, about living your life to the fullest and being all you can be. Patients who end their struggles with eating actually talk about inner harmony and happiness, and many of them rid themselves of depression. That is very spiritual to me.

So you see, weight control isn't about counting calories and starving your body to become thin. Weight and health are about respecting and honoring your body by giving it what it needs to heal, both physically and spiritually.

When you do that, you are truly powerful. Just feeling this way about yourself will raise your quality of life beyond what you had imagined possible.

As one patient, Anna, said, "I was always overweight and felt that my body was letting me down. I now understand that I was letting it down. I now listen to my body, give it what it needs, and it answers by doing what I want. This is the beginning of a beautiful friendship!"

Mantras

You now understand that mantras are mini-meditations used to focus the power of your mind. Used daily, they help concentrate on what you want to achieve, while eliminating thoughts that have held you back in the past. Mantras are extremely powerful tools for growth. Make them part of your daily routine, and watch how success and fulfillment grow—not just for weight management, but in all parts of your life. By now you should know the message of this book. You are realizing:

I have the power to do anything I want.

As you start this program, begin your day by reminding yourself of how to feed your lean body. *I'm becoming thin because I give my lean body protein.*

Every time you eat anything, this mantra should come to mind. You should look at what you're about to eat and ask yourself, "Am I feeding my lean body with this?" This should be your core mantra, just as protein is the trunk of your Food Tree.

Once you realize the true nature of sugar as a toxic additive, you'll recognize sugar for what it is. Your mantra will then be: *This is a metabolic toxin; it's toxic garbage and I don't like it!*

The "I don't like it" part is as important as the "toxic garbage" part. Willpower doesn't work! Besides, it's short-lived. Once your inner computer has registered that you really don't like something, it's a lot easier not to eat it. This is truly changing your mind. It's also the most difficult mantra to get past. It takes persistent practice and repetition to change ingrained patterns that deliver a load of built-in gratification, such as destructive eating.

If you feel as though you've kicked an addiction, you might want to congratulate yourself by saying, "I am clean and sober from sugar."

If you're frustrated when the weight doesn't drop off as quickly as you'd like, you might end up sabotaging yourself with "white-knuckle dieting." Everyone loses weight differently. On your journey toward weight loss, your body sometimes pauses to reshape or shrink mass. Some people get very anxious: "I've sacrificed to lose weight and nothing happened in the last week or two." Not so. Plenty happened. It just didn't register on the scale. And if you sacrificed, there's a problem. Rather than a diet, this is an ongoing process of inventing a new style of eating to turn yourself into a thin person.

The pounds will come off in their own time. Remember: We only stick with something new when we think it's fun. If you decide that a new style of eating is fun, you'll stick with it. The mantra that will anchor this philosophy for you might be: "This is my new style and I'm just having fun!"

If you're not crazy about vegetables, think of them as colors you're adding to your plate:

"Red yellow and green make me healthy and lean." (Some of my patients insist that they're "lean and mean." One was "a lean, mean fighting machine!") Once you add fiber to your protein, you'll be surprised how quickly you fill up. Add the fat, and you have a complete mantra:

"The Food Tree is the new me!" (Who wants to be the old me?)

If you're a reluctant exerciser, maybe this one will get you off the couch:

"Use it to lose it!" (The "lean, mean machine" might work here.)

If you're self-defeating, you might remember that famous commercial line: "I'm worth it!" Because you really are. If you have problems in this department, working with a counselor might prove valuable.

You now have the hang of it, and you can make up your own affirmations as you need them.

CHAPTER 8
Exercise—Learn to Love It!

W hat lowers weight and increases muscle strength, cardiovascular reserve, bone mineral density, and glucose tolerance, elevates mood, rids you of aches, pains, stress, and depression, prevents disability, and allows you to live longer in better health? Exercise!

And where do you find this anti-illness and anti-aging miracle? Anywhere you want to. Scientifically speaking, apart from nutrition, exercise is one of the major modifiable lifestyle characteristics. In practical terms, it means that if we want to live a good life, we have to remember to get off that couch.

Let's start by clearing up a myth around exercise. While it will do all the above wonderful things for you, it won't necessarily make and keep your weight normal.

That myth was created from early exercise studies in which the subjects were fit young men. Life catches up with us. Aging, hormones, and other factors cause metabolic slowdown. We also exercise in spurts. If it takes five days of gym to keep our weight down, we'll eventually "crack," and exercise less—and gain weight. Countless overweight patients have had this experience. Lesson: your proper nutrition has to be in place for exercise to keep you thin.

Others come to me saying, "I exercise every day. I'm in great shape, but I'm not losing weight." They've just performed a one-person clinical experiment reinforcing that weight is basically a function of nutrition. Once I help them change their eating, the pounds come off the exercisers faster and easier than from the sedentary ones. My point is this: If you eat to keep your insulin high, your body will try to hang on to weight even if you eat less and exercise. That's what insulin does for a living, remember?

Exercise speeds up your weight loss and shapes you beautifully as you lose. A toned muscle looks different from a flabby one. Exercise also allows you to eat more in maintenance mode without gaining weight. Feast your eyes again on the above list of all the other things that are in it for you. Activity triggers the compensation mechanism that lowers your blood sugar. And let me make my favorite point: Exercise will change your life. Exercise is like the credit card: priceless. Except the price is right. You can't afford *not* to exercise.

If you exercise in addition to eating your daily requirement of protein, you'll change your body composition and become smaller at a higher weight, because you're preserving the heavier muscle and losing the lighter fat. You'll become thin and muscular. This relationship is well known by athletes, and it's borne out in the Food Tree. Athletes and bodybuilders take this principle to an extreme: they're thin, but heavy. Muscle is working, lean tissue. The more you have and the more you work it, the more energy you burn. This again means that if you're in maintenance mode, you can eat as much sugar as you exercise off.

I tell my patients that they have a daily bank account of food they can draw from. If they withdraw the high numbers (i.e., high glycemic-index sugars), they need to deposit exercise, or their accounts will soon be lopsided, not to say bottom-heavy.

Exercise is any physical activity that raises your heart rate from its resting rate. This is an indication that your metabolism is elevated. You're now working your muscles, including your heart, which is your blood-pumping muscle.

While your muscles get a workout and you lower your blood sugar, exercise influences your other body systems, deposits calcium in your bones, and connects brain-neuron transmitters that regulate mood and stress. The positive metabolic effects spread like wildfire through your entire body. After exercise, your metabolism returns to baseline slowly, and so the positive effects are sustained for hours.

You're now in a positive cycle, because you must continue to exercise to keep your systems toned (or tuned, as it were). How much must you exercise to reap all these benefits? You must get your heart rate up for 30–45 minutes twice a week to maintain, and three times or more to build up your condition. The President's Council on Physical Fitness and Sports recommends that we exercise 60 minutes five times a week.

You can calculate the intensity of your exercise on the following scale: Your maximal heart rate (MHR) = 220 minus your age. Low-intensity exercise is defined as achieving a heart rate of less than 60% of your MHR. Moderate exercise is when you work at a heart rate of 60–80% of MHR. You should not exceed 80% unless you're in a supervised athlete's program. Note that resting heart rate tends to be higher in women (up to 80 beats per minute), and somewhat lower in men (as low as 60 beats per minute).

If you're over thirty-five years old and have been inactive for a long time, or have any kind of cardiovascular disease, get medical clearance before starting exercise. It's fine to start small. In fact, if it's been a long time, you should. I tell my patients to start so minimally that they can't fail. For example, walk for five minutes, and then add more as you feel able to. The point is that you go for it.

Formally, we divide exercise into aerobic and anaerobic training, simply meaning whether you have adequate oxygen when you exercise. Aerobic exercise will condition your heart and muscles; anaerobic exercise will strengthen you.

We have two types of muscle fibers. The slow ones can maximize fat burning at 60–80% of MHR. This is aerobic exercise, meaning there's enough oxygen present. Biochemically, it means that the muscle works slowly enough to break down complex sugars and fat for fuel. At that point, you're still able to talk in full sentences. These muscles are our daily workhorses. Stretching and low weights (up to 8–10 pounds) will tone and work your slow muscle fibers.

Anaerobic exercise implies that there's not enough oxygen present to metabolize fat, and the muscle needs fast food to work (the fast fibers). Heavy weights and more repetitions will recruit those fast, heavy lifters. This is when your body needs quick sugar. Eating a piece of fruit before exercise will help. Even so, your body doesn't utilize this sugar very efficiently without adequate oxygen. If you run out of sugar and get short of breath, you're approaching anaerobe condition and exhaustion. You might have seen runners fall over at the finish line. Or you might have exercised too hard without carbo-loading just beforehand and experienced fatigue or plain exhaustion.

Next we differentiate among endurance (cardiovascular conditioning), flexibility training (stretching), and strength training against resistance. Your exercise program might include cardiovascular exercise with short spurts of high-intensity training to help you recruit all the different muscle fibers and give you time to recover in between. Your warm-up might be the flexibility component. You might hire a personal trainer to set up a program that includes your goals.

On the other hand, if you're getting started, you might simply start walking, biking, or swimming, the three most all-round forms of aerobic or cardiovascular conditioning. A couple of hand weights will work your upper body, and a few heavy lifts will recruit your fast fiber for balance. You might work out a 5–10 minute stretching routine to start off and to cool down.

The important thing is that you get started doing some form of exercise. Pick something you like and tailor it to your personality.

Exercise is cumulative. Even if you do only one of the above, but incorporate it into your daily activities for fifteen minutes at a time, it counts toward your goal. Your best starting point is to make it part of your lifestyle. Resolve to walk to the store instead of driving, or park your car far away from wherever you're going, and take the stairs instead of the elevator.

Some people like to exercise alone. A treadmill at home or a walk in the neighborhood might be a start. Others need company and music to get going. Your style would be a gym. Some do best with a trainer. Also, are you a morning or night person? Don't make it complicated or theoretical. We moved around for thousands of years without knowing how many calories we burned per hour. On the other hand, if numbers interest or motivate you, see the table on page 132 for energy expenditures of the most common daily activities. Do something during the week, and then expand on it over the weekend. Have you ever used the hiking trails in your neighborhood? That might be a great discovery. You don't need to be an athlete to select an activity that's appropriate for you and that you enjoy. As with proper eating, you just need to find your fun.

I'll share my story with you for inspiration: I hated to exercise in school because it was always about being good at some indoor sport or working on equipment like the gymnasts you see on TV. I was miserable at both, and my gym teacher was the very image of a Prussian army general. I loathed this woman who made me fail at everything. Meanwhile, I loved hiking and skiing. Fast-forward to medical school, where I was invited to join an aerobics class. I wryly said, "I don't *do* gym." My friend insisted, dragged me along, and there it was—the music, the wonderful instructor, and the camaraderie, something purely fun that I could do. I discovered one of my lifelong passions, aerobics! It's truly my most important source of therapy, physical as well as mental. I have a whole new outlook when I leave the gym. What if I'd never given it a chance?

If you find a passion, the way I found aerobics, the habit comes by itself. If I don't get to class for a couple of weeks, I feel sick. Feeling that way, and knowing how great I'll feel after exercising, drives me back there.

It's rare to fall instantly in love with any form of activity; you have to give it time and develop a habit around it. So how do we develop a habit? It's less complicated than eating, but it hinges on developing a pattern, which again is nothing but brain reprogramming. The reprogramming for exercise is a matter of incorporating it into your schedule in the form of an unbreakable weekly date. You schedule it as a priority at a certain time on a certain day, making it a must-do appointment.

In the beginning it might be a chore, but as you begin to feel and look better, it becomes a positive reinforcement situation that drives you back to it again and again. Make a commitment to have it on your schedule for a month, and make it positive.

You might use the carrot-on-the-stick principle: you can only watch your favorite TV show from the treadmill, or listen to your favorite music if you take a walk. Anchoring the exercise habit works on the same principles any change does: information messenger and recipient.

How do you message to yourself about exercise? Hopefully not by saying, "sedentary is beautiful." Remember that sedentary is dangerous to your health. I have a patient who's built his entire program of change on "I'm a lean, mean machine." If you're a woman, you might want to focus on something less macho. "Use it or lose it" is a favorite mantra. Think about what motivates you about exercise and create your own affirmation around it. And then use it to focus your exercise energy.

When it comes to exercise, we often have role models, but they tend to be elite athletes and remote from our own reality. However much we cheer them on from the armchair, vicarious exercise doesn't work. That leaves us with the messengers of our own environment. Do you see yourself jogging through your neighborhood in tights and headphones? Maybe that's not where you want to begin. Look around you and think who might be interested in starting at your level. Recruit a friend or neighbor or a whole group to walk at a certain time every week. Mall walking is popular in some cities.

Perhaps the stated purpose of a social club you belong to could include an activity such as walking. If your meetings include food, you could do two in one: first go walking, then finish by sharing the "treat of the week"—a creative, healthy snack or meal. This would get you out there, and could inspire people who otherwise wouldn't get started on their own.

In a bad mood? Studies show that exercise is a very powerful antidote to depression. In fact, some studies suggest that exercise is equal to medications in some cases of mood disorder. My experience with overweight patients is that many of them are depressed about their weight and health. They tell me so straight out. Once they change that, their depression improves or goes away entirely.

Vanity is a very good thing. Exercise makes you snazzy-looking while you become thin. Snazzy is good. It's also another word for sexy.

Obesity adds twenty years to your body, including your heart. And you don't feel so great either. People express it as "I've lost my edge." Along with eating right, there's no better anti-aging therapy than exercise. Studies confirm this time and again. This combination will give you back your edge, I promise. And the price for this therapy is a lot less than most anti-aging potions.

You now have the inside scoop on the formula for anti-aging. Curiously, it coincides with the philosophy of this book.

Low calories, low sugar, moderate exercise.

Please beware: Apart from diets, anti-aging is the next fertile ground for scamming. Fortunately there is one recent discovery of exciting scientific merit: Brain plasticity. This roughly means that our brains keep ever changing and learning for as long as we live. Therefore by doing certain mental exercises combined with physical activity, we can rejuvenate our brain function by some ten years. There won't be a pill to achieve this kind of vitality real soon. Neither will there be one for looking like you eat right.

Will I see you on the trail this weekend?

CHAPTER 9
Adopt a Food Tree

Y ou can now see that overweight is how our bodies put us on notice that our nutrition isn't keeping us in our G-I window. We can deny it and take pills, potions, and remedies, which, scientifically, is equivalent to insisting that the earth is flat. It will never be flat, and our bodies will not be normal till we accept the facts of nutrition.

You've seen that your body—the magnificent machine—operates on basic biochemical principles, and that food is metabolized accordingly. Let's summarize those principles.

When we eat, the body writes a glucose-insulin curve over time. This curve decides our weight. It also decides our health. Key to both is keeping our curve inside the glucose-insulin window.

Weight loss or weight gain happens right after meals, and depends on the composition of the meal. Too much sugar drives the curve into weight gain. The swift changes in blood sugar make us hungry and perpetuate this curve on an addiction principle. Lowering the curve with protein and fiber gets us off the addiction curve by coding for weight loss and fullness. Carbohydrates are sugars in many guises, from the good to the bad to the ugly. It's crucial that we recognize which ones have food value and which are "unfermented alcohol," and respect them the way we respect alcohol: potentially toxic substances if we abuse them.

Protein is the stuff of life. All sorts of regulatory body functions are carried out through protein. In fact, insulin itself is made of protein. It lowers the G-I curve and codes for fullness.

We need to eat our daily requirement of biologically complete proteins to maintain a strong lean body.

Behind the scenes, fat runs the show. It comes in many forms, some of them crucial to good health. Fat is a basic part of all cell membranes and cellular functions, and remember: it's the precursor of the super-hormones that code for whether our body is in a state of inflammation and what kind of health we're in. The right fats keep us out of inflammation; the wrong ones contribute to aches and pains, metabolic illnesses, and a host of inflammatory reactions we might not even recognize as such.

The main regulator of this cascade is our old friend insulin.

Cholesterol is the specialist. It's necessary for healthy cells and many hormones and enzymes. It supports our brain and nervous system. It appears in atherosclerotic lesions in arteries, and has thus gotten a bad rap. When we eat badly and gain weight, cholesterol is overproduced and becomes a problem. If we eat according to the principles of the body (maintain low insulin), cholesterol is normally not a problem but a necessary building block.

Do you notice the common denominator in all the rules of healthy body biochemistry? *Low insulin, of course.*

We've Taken Nutrition Full Circle

You now understand that high sugar causes high insulin, which causes bad super-hormones, which causes inflammation illness and sugar addiction, which causes more sugar consumption and so on. And you've seen that the G-I curve is the root of all metabolic good and evil in your body because it determines what sort of super-hormones you make.

If you learn nothing else from this book, remember that the first and last rule of the body is to keep insulin low at all costs. Everything else will follow. And that's the one rule we break and pay for all the time.

This information is enough to get many people out of their bad-health ruts and start new and different lives for themselves. But often there's more to eating, and it might not be as easy to rein in as simply understanding the biochemistry of nutrition. Complicating factors may show up in the way we connect food with emotions. It might be anything from bad habits to genetically determined addiction. People who are addicted to sugar often come to see it themselves. Unfortunately it isn't recognized by society. Worse yet, it isn't prevented, it is encouraged—it is everywhere you look!

Visualize It and It Will Happen!

While that's not really true, it is true that we can clear our minds of baggage that stops us getting what we want, including losing weight and overcoming sugar addiction.

It's a matter of recognizing self-defeating patterns, and learning to adapt positive ones. The short version is summarized in something called the Law of Attraction of Energy. I've used this principle for ten years, simply because it works. It's an integral part of the Food Tree.

Make no mistake about it: The best way to address addiction is to prevent it!

Tried and True

The Food Tree is based on the collective body of medical research as well as my decade of experience as a physician helping thousands of people—including those "hopeless" cases who have come to my door as a last resort. These include stay-at-home moms and couch-potato dads, lonely hearts and socialites, doctors and other medical professionals, older folks, and super athletes—and even so-called nutrition gurus who've secretly sought out my advice to control their own weight.

The Food Tree is evidence based. Its principles agree with emerging medical literature and yield consistent, reproducible results.

We can eat healthily; people do. We can make food more interesting and varied than our ancestors ever could. We just need to reconnect with our long-suffering bodies and start liking what they like, and we'll see a beautiful friendship!

What I share here wasn't available to me when I was young and overweight, struggling to make peace with food. I didn't find my answer in the cola diet, the cabbage diet, the egg-white diet, the grapefruit diet, the starvation diet, or any other of the crazes I desperately tried. The Food Tree is not just another stop on the diet train to nowhere. It is the final station, where you get off the train and end your struggle with the fads.

Your Lean Body Has Been Kept in the Closet!

Your lean, healthy body has been locked in the closet all along, waiting for you to allow it to come to expression. You can do it starting now!

I've shown you that nutrition is the basis for most illnesses seen in modern medical practice. You are an informed person who understands that you're stuck in a struggle, saddling your body with metabolic poisons for food. Your mind calls them treats, but your body is slowly dying from their toxic effects. Look at yourself. Is your body cringing in pain, begging you to stop this abuse?

Our interpretation of the good life has turned into a health nightmare.

A nurse said to me "I'd like to do your program, but I can't give up my carbs." She forgot that it's not my program, it's how her body works. She epitomizes the addicted who won't seek help. I would simply educate her to understand the keys to good health. She remains the perennial victim because she can't face this fact of life.

"But I have to eat." Of course we do. We're just confused. Food doesn't addict us, toxins do. We're being held hostage by a culture that should inform and help us. The consequences are staggering. Inundated with gurus and potions, we don't figure out how it all works. We look for miracles. We're besieged by high-tech, high-priced body measurements of "essential vitamins." We're deluded into thinking the problem is lack of the latest advertised vitamin X, so we spend a fortune on tests, supplements, and nature doctors to administer them to us. Have you noticed that nothing much happens to your weight, blood pressure, diabetes, or whatever problem you're trying to address? Patients come to me with stacks of unnecessary test results from high-priced clinics, and supplements that have impacted nothing but their wallets.

No amount of supplementation or pills will take your body out of inflammation and heal it. But I promise you: When you eat guided by the Food Tree, you unleash a long, complicated chain of biochemical reactions that ends with good super-hormones and wellness for you instead of illness. You are constantly cleansing your body of inflammation and strengthening your defense mechanisms.

This is science, not vitamin retail. It's the best, most affordable health insurance you'll ever have, because all you have to do to be well is eat well.

You now have two choices: You can continue the old way, or you can change.

The old way includes the miracle diet, the new wonder supplement or medication, the quick-fix willpower trip, all of which leave you more powerless and victimized by the wonder gurus.

If you choose change, you now have the opportunity to pack some real power into your life. The first step is to let go of the old and allow something new to happen.

Think of it this way: Change isn't as difficult as it is different. You already have the information. Now you need to use it. Instead of listening to whoever sells you cookies or wants to perform $500 worth of "vitamin" tests on you, ask your body what it wants to eat and start listening. Listen to your body for two weeks and watch what happens.

Watch your energy and mood soar and your weight shrink along with your medication use. Your social life and your sex life might improve as well (that happens a lot!), and you'll spend your money on fun things.

Treat your body as well as you would treat yourself.

Treat your body to the Food Tree.

Visualize the tree. It brings you into balance. You can bring your weight up or down by changing your setpoint. It's easy to visualize, understand, and do.

Instead of crashing at full speed toward the next diet burn, the Food Tree will show you how to create a program for restoring your health naturally. You don't need to be a foodie or a master chef to do this. Basic foods are the best. To start eating well, all you need is a good shopping list and a refrigerator. You have the refrigerator. I give you the food list and show you some basics of simple food preparation (see appendices).

You'll discover that you fill up faster and, that you never need to be hungry, and that food is tasty and exciting. You'll also find that when your body gets building blocks instead of garbage, your quality of life will soar long before the weight comes off. You might not remember having felt so good, because you might not recognize feeling normal. All this time you thought feeling sluggish and tired was the best you could do.

Remember: There's no evidence that our forebears cursed their fate because they didn't have chocolate cake with ice cream. But there's plenty of evidence that obese people suffer malnutrition despite all they eat.

An Active Lifestyle Is an Asset

Let's sum up the broader definition of weight and health: It's a biochemical balance of what we think and eat and how we move. Once out of this balance, we suffer. This means that an active lifestyle is part of the overall picture. Many of us are out of touch with exercise, and it hurts us. Exercise can be learned. The suggestions in chapter 8 can get you started.

Anti-aging? You bet!

This is no idle advertisement. It has been proven over and over again that the fast track to keeping you young goes through: 1) Lowering your caloric intake; 2) Getting the sugar out of your nutrition, and; 3) Exercising moderately. That is the Food Tree.

Once you have all the elements of the program in place, you're now on an anti-aging track. It's the cheapest anti-aging miracle of all, and yet it's priceless.

If All Else Fails, Hire A Coach

Lifestyle coaches are all the rage. We might want to change certain things in our lives, but we get sidetracked and lose our focus, leaving us with a dream that never becomes reality. It's beneficial to have a person who helps us keep centered on what we want to accomplish. Lifestyle coaches do just that. They help us turn our dreams into reality by setting up plans with timelines and concrete steps to get there. It doesn't mean we lack ability, it simply means we need help to prioritize better. In the end, coaches help us do what we come to them and tell them we want to do.

If you can't find the focus to follow the Food Tree, hire a coach to help you. The payoff will be reflected in every aspect of your life.

We're All In This Together

The truth is, of course, that the Food Tree is not just for "dieters." The reason we fail at weight loss and maintenance is that we, as a culture, have been thrown into a complicated addiction that we can't easily get out of. Don't smile—you're next! We don't recognize this simple principle: We're in this together and we can only get out together. We need to beat our sugar addiction together because we're simply too addicted to get out alone. It's not about "them" but about "us." This is a neglected aspect of weight and health, but awareness of it is growing at the moment. It is so important that I've devoted the entire last chapter to it.

Adopt A Food Tree

I've laid out everything for you: how to shop, what to keep in your refrigerator, how to set up your Food Tree, how to think, and how to avoid the pitfalls. The next chapter even shows you how to involve your environment.

We can change our health and transform our lives. Knowledge is power. Create a better life for you and your family and friends—for all your loved ones. Adopt a Food Tree! Do it together. Your school, your church, and your community can all benefit from this plan. Form a Food Tree club with your friends. If they're unwilling to change, let them sit at the bar while you go looking for people who aspire to more.

The reason you should involve your environment is simple: The chances of your succeeding increases dramatically, as do the chances of those who join you. I see this all the time in my practice: patients who have support in their environment do better than those who don't.

As a society, we've lost control over our health and nutrition, and are spiraling downward fast. But we can take back control. We don't need some overweight, medication-chomping politician with better health insurance than we have, and the sugar lobby in his back pocket, to tell us how to live. We can stop being the patient-victims and reclaim control of our health and our quality of life. We can be a positive force in our community and part of the solution.

You certainly can, you've already taken the first step in reading this book.

If you need help, please visit www.FoodTreeMD.com

CHAPTER 10
We're All In This Together

You might have recognized yourself many times throughout this book, because most of us are in it. You now have all the information and insight you'll need to change your life, and I hope you will. But too many of us will end up like the mythical Sisyphus, forever rolling that boulder up the hills of Hades, only to have it crash down again. It isn't five pounds—it's often the entire boulder!

You also appreciate why that's so. You've seen it in words and graphs: we've created an environment that doesn't accommodate people who want to eat real food, and that's so conducive to sugar addiction that all of us are becoming addicted!

A surgeon I know started using the Food Tree, but gave up early on, saying, "I can't find the foods I need in the hospital, and my schedule doesn't permit it." She really put her finger squarely on the problem: "The real world just doesn't function like this." That includes the hospital.

No kidding. Listen to the woman who said, "My blood sugar turned out to be normal—I can go back to eating mashed potatoes and dessert!" She might just as well be saying, "My liver is still holding up—I can go back to drinking!"

That sums up how we think as a culture and why we can't stop the onslaught of obesity.

We suffer this self-inflicted, opportunistic addiction because we unwittingly invited it in, and now we're unable to tame it. How long will the crisis continue? Until we're willing to accept the truth—and more important, until we're willing to change it.

Drinking was once thought glamorous. This seems shocking now. When we realized that alcohol was a toxic substance creating massive health problems, we started informing people and warning them against it. We even enacted legislation and offered treatment options and support to kick the habit.

Cigarettes were all the rage till the long-term results of smoking could no longer be ignored. Now we all know that smoking is dangerous to your health. It's strongly discouraged and restricted. We changed the tide when the information got so compelling that we could no longer plead ignorance.

The difference is that we changed as a society, not because we told individuals to lay off tobacco and alcohol while we advertised it to them and served it everywhere, but because we put our integrity as a society behind the warnings.

When it comes to sugar, the information has not been forthcoming, and the willingness has been in short supply. Here's the short list of why we compromise our integrity:

"We're Not Sure Sugar is That Bad for Us!"

In 2003, the World Health Organization proposed a campaign to reduce sugar intake by 10 percent. The US sugar lobby promptly squelched it. "We don't really know that sugar is that bad for us!" Meanwhile, we continue our long, painful suicide, living in a sugar-induced haze, while the monster is at our door. Twenty percent of the federal budget goes to funding Medicare/Medicaid. Forty percent of health dollars are spent on type 2 diabetes alone—an unnecessary illness. These numbers are ballooning by the day due to lifestyle illnesses of the baby-boomer generation. Statistically, boomers are in no position to finance their own retirement, let alone buy their own healthcare or ever more expensive lifestyle medications. My years in primary care confirm these numbers. Up to 70 percent of the patients I saw did not have to be patients— they just needed to change their lifestyles. The health-restoring results of removing sugar and balancing our nutrition fulfill the criteria of evidence-based medicine: They are reproducible anytime, anywhere. Are we sure yet?

"How do we know it will work?"

"We need more studies." This is an obstructionist argument. We already have more studies. We also have proof that nutrition works. It has worked since the beginning of time, long before all the lifestyle medications were invented. We didn't need to take medications to survive. We're just living on a cloud while the sugar is hitting the fan.

"Our economy would suffer greatly."

This seems to suggest that it's not suffering as it is! If the economy of this great country depends on keeping our people ill and dying prematurely, maybe it's time to rethink our economy. I haven't heard that it's about to tank due to lackluster cigarette sales. I also doubt it would collapse from low junk-food sales. But I know that our economy is bulging at the seams from the cost of obesity. I also know for sure that the entrepreneurial spirit of this country would respond to any changes we make to move business successfully to where it needs to go next!

We Need to Belong

Why do group dieters agree to count calories and go to bed hungry? Why inflict pain by piercing one's nipples? Why do members of religious sects agree to commit suicide? Psychology 101 tells us that we need to belong to something greater than ourselves, and if we find "our group" we're willing to do whatever they do to be part of it. Visit a Japanese restaurant and you'll see this principle at work in a most positive sense. When they bring you a slice of orange for dessert, you find it delightfully refreshing. You don't ask to see the dessert tray, because you're in an environment that would make you feel out of place if you did. The larger your group, the more likely each individual is to succeed. The Japanese culture as a group was virtually free of cardiac disease until it became westernized. This opens up the possibility of turning all this group-oriented energy into a culture of healthy diners with creatively reinvented dessert trays.

Where are Our Role Models?—We're Too Addicted to Get Out Alone

We all want to be in the right group. It's called being "in." Who's in? The leaders and the majority of our group. They know what to wear, what to do, and what to eat. They don't smoke in public and are very careful about their alcohol use. But they readily flaunt their junk food, and if that's having fun, why should I have to suffer through my boring food and perhaps have to endure their comments on my "diet food?" I actually had a teen patient who had to defer learning her Food Tree until summer vacation because doing it singled her out in a negative way.

You can now see why we fail and our leaders shun their responsibility; why we crack in maintenance mode, and why weight-loss experts aren't necessarily any thinner or healthier than their patients. We don't want to sacrifice. We want to do what everyone else does. If I see you modeling the good life by being fat and unhealthy, I want it too. Imagine trying to be sober in a society where everyone drinks six to eleven servings of alcohol per meal, by decree of health experts! And wherever you go, everyone sells, buys, and drinks alcohol as the mainstay of their nutrition, calling it food. Grotesque, you say?

Walk down the street and look at the names of "coffee bars." Notice how many have names that include "sugar/sweet/cake/cookie." My husband wryly remarked, "I'm waiting for 'the Glycemic Index Café' to arrive." Sugar addicts live in such an all-tavern society! They're enabled everywhere, but find no support to become clean and sober. The grocery store, the restaurant, the vending machine, and the family dinner table—these are the taverns of a sugar addict. If you want to fit in and have fun, you must eat sugar. As long as food is "deprivation" and sugar is "good," we can't change.

As long as we don't recognize that we're in this together and need to clean up together, we're powerless to change.

"They" Won't Do It

This is true as long as it's about "them." We tend to abstract this whole pesky issue by telling our kids what to do. We also pick "people who need to go on a diet," making them different while we're medicating our own high cholesterol. Did it ever occur to you that if we all ate "different," then different would be "regular," and the sugar eater would be different? You get it: We all need to become "different," the sooner the better. The truth is that this isn't about *them,* it's about *us.*

How Can We Change All This?

Declare war on the right enemy. We've ranted against fat for decades, and even invented virtual fat and fat blockers while we increased the sugar in the fat-free products. Many of us made the change, but the results were disappointing because fat wasn't the main culprit; we only became more addicted to sugar. Most people can change to using olive oil and trim the fat off meats. Changing from sugar to low-GI carbs is another matter.

We are dealing with an epidemic addiction and suffering the ravages of sugar much like we suffered the ravages of alcohol before prohibition.

We need a temperance movement, only the mothers are addicted! If you could give your child the best, would you? What kind of health are you giving your child?

We All Need to Be Informed about Sugar

This will take a massive education campaign. Eliminating soda from vending machines in schools is just another overbearing gesture and doesn't explain anything to anyone. Replacing them with fruit juice at the same GI only speaks to our ignorance. We need to accept the biochemical facts and agree on what sugar is. Only then can we relegate it to where it belongs. The food industry gives us "what we want" because we don't know what we want. We have to educate ourselves and change "what we want." Remember the old ad "This is your brain on drugs?" We need a "This is your pancreas on sugar" commercial to inform people.

Zero Tolerance for the Sugar Lobby

We need to stop supporting people and companies that manipulate us into thinking that sugary, fat-laden processed things are food. This is also a tough one. Our legislators fall down on so many other public-interest issues because of the corruptive nature of the lobbying system. Governor Huckabee has called attention to obesity in Arkansas by his leadership. To his credit, he has changed his lifestyle, but showing people your diet isn't enough to turn the tide. Once people see the pizza commercial, the governor's new lifestyle isn't reinforced, but contradicted. We deserve a break today—from manipulative messages about sugar! We have to stop tolerating policies that undermine our health, and demand that sugar come off television the way alcohol and cigarettes have.

As part of our campaign against cigarettes and alcohol, we removed all ads from view, and then we taxed their use to emphasize that this was nothing we needed. Now that you realize sugar is not a food, the idea of taxing it might not be so bad. The sugar tax could be funneled into education and incentives for the food industry to bring us appealing, affordable alternatives.

The sugar industry spends $11 billion annually encouraging your child to eat sugar! This will come as no surprise to you if you monitor what your children watch on TV. The reason is: "We don't know that sugar is bad for you." Remember that one? It might be time for you to write your government representative and demand that this proven metabolic toxin be treated like the others under the law. No child needs to eat any manmade sugar product. If we did need to, we'd have died out 100,000 years ago. When she was growing up, my mother didn't have available to her any of the products we're talking about. She's ninety-four years old.

End the tyranny of the medico-pharmaceutical complex. This industry is fueling medical practice by advertising drugs and indoctrinating physicians in their use at the expense of lifestyle considerations. Lifestyle is actually snickered at in most medical seminars. Research confirms that doctors show arrogance and prejudice against overweight people and the doctors who treat them.

The bombardment on TV of the different medications that you should ask your doctor for is deplorable, and should be exchanged for taking initiative and demanding information on how to avoid them.

Promote healthy foods the way we now promote sugar. For years we've subsidized the sugar industry. We're betting on the wrong horse and losing. First of all, we need to recognize food when we see it. We need to move our misplaced subsidies toward making the food industry grow and sell food, not sugar. We also need to make food competitive with sugar for the consumer, or sugar will win every time anyone with limited budget and information stands in the cafeteria line. To get people out of the fast-food outlets, we need to teach people how to shop and eat, starting in grade school. My younger patients who eat according to the Food Tree can't eat in school cafeterias because what's served there is mostly sugar laced with fat! Hospital food is equally abysmal—short on nutrition and long on fillers and not very health promoting. Even good restaurants resort to the perennial bed of mashed potatoes to serve as the main vegetable. Why? Because you don't protest.

Promote good health the way we now promote ill health. Incentives are positive reinforcement, and they work! There are several proven incentives. Let's start with a big one:

Money. Appealing to our wallets is extremely effective. People who don't need to clip coupons simply do because they're available. Ten percent off is a big draw, though we might not really know what the price was before. Business knows this and uses it all the time because it works. It's in our nature to want a bargain. This means there's an entire untapped pool of people who'd like a discount on anything, including their healthcare. This tool should be put to use. People should be given financial incentives along with the means to change.

Since the obesity-related burden on the medical system tops our charts, we should change our priorities to gear the medical system decisively toward rewarding preventive medicine, starting with nutrition. This would make us individual stockholders in our own health. Unfortunately, our system doesn't give the patient an option, and rewards physicians for keeping chronic patients exactly that, not for helping them get well.

The insurance industry is bitterly opposed to paying for or creating incentives around weight and nutrition issues, because "diets" don't work. As we've seen by now, "dieters" don't change the culture—information does. Yet, curiously, insurance companies agree to pay for all the complications of obesity to the tune of near-bankruptcy.

Now that we understand nutrition, we can work with information. If nutrition were taught to us, and if normal weight, blood pressure, blood sugar, and cholesterol translated into rebates on health insurance, we might see a surge of healthy eaters. The numbers in my office suggest that if taught the Food Tree, up to 30 percent of chronic patients in diabetic and metabolic clinics would become non-patients in a few months. Adding incentives could make the numbers rise quickly.

When people rid themselves of up to ten medications, it's a discount to the patient, and, over time, an incredible savings to their employer as well as to the healthcare system. This should be rewarded by discounts on health insurance.

Time. This is the other important incentive we should take seriously. In this work ethic of loyalty points for long hours, people work those ten-hour days and go home to another job—chores and child-care—leaving them overwhelmed, frustrated, and unhealthy. While we've come a long way since the industrial revolution, the work ethic that straps individuals this way and destroys their health is much more insidious now.

I've seen many patients like Bob, a hard-driving business professional who came to me overweight and ill, clearly borrowing against his future. He shed some thirty pounds, improving his health dramatically. He was looking to include exercise, but had to give up, caught in the lifestyle of "the high-end trap." I find it difficult to remind this type of patient about the benefits of exercise. The corporate chant is, "We can't afford shorter hours." But can we afford the ill health and loss of productivity we're creating? Compared to our European counterparts who work shorter hours, both our productivity and health are lagging, which suggests that all this devotion to company time may be counterproductive.

Role Models and Leadership

In response to recent research it has been suggested that obesity is a "contagious social illness." Do you see what I see? *Obesity is learned. That means thinness is learned too.*

The first and strongest role model you meet in life is a parent. This person makes executive decisions about what you do and eat for all the habit-forming years of your life. If you're in this very powerful position, what do you message to your child? Remember: children live by the mantra "Why should I do what you say when I can see how you live?" Knowing what you now know, you're in a position to give your child the priceless gift of good health. But it starts with you. Do you "diet" and send your child out to eat fast food? Or do you put your child on a "diet" while the rest of the family wallows in sugar? Don't laugh—many people do. Do you recognize that with every fast-food meal, your child gets an entire day's worth of calories in one meal but very little nutrition? You're sending your child to a tavern. Is this really what you want? With relatively small changes in our behavior we could role model what's right and create a culture full of fine diners.

I recently helped a mother change habits. She used to buy fast food. She now buys easy fixings: ready-roasted chicken, simple cuts of meat or fish for grilling, prepared stir-fries, and washed lettuce and veggies.

Guess what? Her whole family shows up at dinnertime, they've all lost weight, and, according to the patient, "My family loves it!"

Bringing her teenage daughter to me, an overweight mother said, "She needs to lose weight." This woman was messaging that she expected her daughter to do something she didn't think she could do herself.

The "cool people" in social groups pick up fashion cues. No one needs to tell women what shape their handbags must be this year. The mantra is: "This is what all the cool people wear." We need to get the cool people to be role models for good nutrition, starting with our California governor. He has taken great interest in physical fitness, which is wonderful. I challenge him to make broccoli as trendy as cigars. I challenge all our leaders to stop fretting and show the vision and courage to lead

It is amazing that it takes a study in the *New England Journal of Medicine* to remind us that role modeling works for better or for worse. When it comes to weight and health, worse has won out by some 70 percent. It's not going to change unless we make it happen.

Hollywood is full of role models, many of them civic minded. They stood up against cigarettes and alcohol. It's not cool anymore to smoke in California. They'd surely pitch in against sugar. This message might even be close to their hearts, since they already live by it.

Hollywood and Madison Avenue message. They create trends and positive mantras to get us to do what they want. They do it by uplifting rather than depressing us. We should take their cues. "The Food Tree is cool!" sure beats "You need to go on a diet."

Everyone Should Learn the Food Tree

Balanced nutrition—not the USDA Food Pyramid—should be taught in schools. It should also be taught to those of us who are out of school. Everyone should know what happens to their body when they eat well and what happens when they eat poorly. Everyone should understand the almost-linear relationship between their nutrition and use of lifestyle medications.

We, Not "They," Need to Change

You might not have thought about it before, but you now realize that it's basic mass psychology: The social aspect of obesity is what created this crisis. People respond to their environment, for better or for worse. That includes you, and me, and them. That's the reason we have an epidemic of obesity and bad health. Recent research is finally looking at this and confirming it. If we fail to recognize and tackle this problem, history will see us as pathetic rather than powerful. We can do so much better.

We're all in this together. We can get out together.

APPENDICES
Tables and Charts

As a general rule, if you're a patient, work with your doctor on any changes to your nutrition, because your medications will most likely need to be adjusted.

	Normal						Overweight					Obese				
BMI	19	20	21	22	23	24	25	26	27	28	29	30	31	32	33	34
Height (Feet/Inches)	Body Weight (Pounds)															
4'10"	91	96	100	105	110	115	119	124	129	134	138	143	148	153	158	162
4'11"	94	99	104	109	114	119	124	128	133	138	143	148	153	158	163	168
5'0"	97	102	107	112	118	123	128	133	138	143	148	153	158	163	168	174
5'1"	100	106	111	116	122	127	132	137	143	148	153	158	164	169	174	180
5'2"	104	109	115	120	126	131	136	142	147	153	158	164	169	175	180	186
5'3"	107	113	118	124	130	135	141	146	152	158	163	169	175	180	186	191
5'4"	110	116	122	128	134	140	145	151	157	163	169	174	180	186	192	197
5'5"	114	120	126	132	138	144	150	156	162	168	174	180	186	192	198	204
5'6"	118	124	130	136	142	148	155	161	167	173	179	186	192	198	204	210
5'7"	121	127	134	140	146	153	159	166	172	178	185	191	198	204	211	217
5'8"	125	131	138	144	151	158	164	171	177	184	190	197	203	210	216	223
5'9"	128	135	142	149	155	162	169	176	182	189	196	203	209	216	223	230
5'10"	132	139	146	153	160	167	174	181	188	195	202	209	216	222	229	236
5'11"	136	143	150	157	165	172	179	186	193	200	208	215	222	229	236	243
6'0"	140	147	154	162	169	177	184	191	199	206	213	221	228	235	242	250
6'1"	144	151	159	166	174	182	189	197	204	212	219	227	235	242	250	257
6'2"	148	155	163	171	179	186	194	202	210	218	225	233	241	249	256	264
6'3"	152	160	168	176	184	192	200	208	216	224	232	240	248	256	264	272
6'4"	156	164	172	180	189	197	205	213	221	230	238	246	254	263	271	279

Source: Adapted from *Clinical Guidelines on the Identification, Evaluation, and Treatment of Overweight and Obesity in Adults: The Evidence Report.*

Extreme Obesity																				BMI
35	36	37	38	39	40	41	42	43	44	45	46	47	48	49	50	51	52	53	54	
Body Weight (Pounds)																				Height (Feet/Inches)
167	172	177	181	186	191	196	201	205	210	215	220	224	229	234	239	244	248	253	258	4'10"
173	178	183	188	193	198	203	208	212	217	222	227	232	237	242	247	252	257	262	267	4'11"
179	184	189	194	199	204	209	215	220	225	230	235	240	245	250	255	261	266	271	276	5'0"
185	190	195	201	206	211	217	222	227	232	238	243	248	254	259	264	269	275	280	285	5'1"
191	196	202	207	213	218	224	229	235	240	246	251	256	262	267	273	278	284	289	295	5'2"
197	203	208	214	220	225	231	237	242	248	254	259	265	270	278	282	287	293	299	304	5'3"
204	209	215	221	227	232	238	244	250	256	262	267	273	279	285	291	296	302	308	314	5'4"
210	216	222	228	234	240	246	252	258	264	270	276	282	288	294	300	306	312	318	324	5'5"
216	223	229	235	241	247	253	260	266	272	278	284	291	297	303	309	315	322	328	334	5'6"
223	230	236	242	249	255	261	268	274	280	287	293	299	306	312	319	325	331	338	344	5'7"
230	236	243	249	256	262	269	276	282	289	295	302	308	315	322	328	335	341	348	354	5'8"
236	243	250	257	263	270	277	284	291	297	304	311	318	324	331	338	345	351	358	365	5'9"
243	250	257	264	271	278	285	292	299	306	313	320	327	334	341	348	355	362	369	376	5'10"
250	257	265	272	279	286	293	301	308	315	322	329	338	343	351	358	365	372	379	386	5'11"
258	265	272	279	287	294	302	309	316	324	331	338	346	353	361	368	375	383	390	397	6'0"
265	272	280	288	295	302	310	318	325	333	340	348	355	363	371	378	386	393	401	408	6'1"
272	280	287	295	303	311	319	326	334	342	350	358	365	373	381	389	396	404	412	420	6'2"
279	287	295	303	311	319	327	335	343	351	359	367	375	383	391	399	407	415	423	431	6'3"
287	295	304	312	320	328	336	344	353	361	369	377	385	394	402	410	418	426	435	443	6'4"

This chart is only a guideline. Your optimal weight will vary with your body frame, body type, and how muscular you are. Using the Food Tree, you'll typically end up with more muscle, weighing a little over your "ideal" weight as shown here, and clock in at a BMI closer to 25. This is especially true for men, since the BMI charts are unisex, and men naturally have larger muscle mass than women. Most athletes are muscular and are invariably heavier than their "ideal" BMI.

Your Protein Requirements

In Maintenance Mode: your "ideal" body weight in pounds × .45 grams
In Weight-loss Mode: your "ideal" body weight in pounds × .7 grams
Add 10% for nursing, 20% for pregnancy.
Add 10% for light activity, up to 30% for hard physical activity.

Athletes have special requirements; their nutrition must be calculated on an individual basis.

About The Glycemic Index

The Glycemic Index is a numerical rating of carbohydrates denoting how fast and high they raise blood sugar and insulin (see the G-I curve, chapter 2). The given number is based on eating enough of a carbohydrate to supply 50 grams of sugar. Fifty grams of glucose tops the scale at 100. Well, not really, since maltose (in malt, beer) is two glucose molecules bound together and breaks the scale at a whopping 105! On the other hand, fructose raises insulin very mildly, and registers at about 23. Legumes and berries and dairy rate in the 20s–30s. But look what happens when you mash beans. Vegetables aren't studied individually because, as green beans suggest, you can't eat enough of them to harm yourself. Think of them as low (less than 40).

Fruits are medium (40–50) and to be respected. For instance, an apple or a pear gives you nutrition and fiber at GI around 10. A pound will bring your GI to around 40. Half a pound of bananas will jack your GI up to 60. Now look at cereal: 3 ounces and you're at 85! A whole quart of milk or yogurt will be around 30, but add sugar and suddenly the meter starts ticking! Ice cream, yogurt, and chocolate may vary in sugar/fat content, so their GIs may vary.

Grains and sugars, the toxic cousins, are above 50 (high) and it takes very little to get there. Note that pasta has lower GI than most grain products because it contains eggs as a stabilizer, but it doesn't take much to raise GI. The toxicity of carbs is like that of alcohol: there's no magic number, but you know when you've had enough. When your waistband is unhappy, so is your whole body. Grains and pasta vary depending on starch type and content. Milling, mashing, and cooking increase GI. Averages are given. The GI of grains is academic unless they're eaten as cereals or milled for use in baking.

What nutrients come from sugars and milled grains? Not many, unless they've been added. Now take a second look at your breakfast roll. Pale, sticky, and pasty, actually worse that that: it's the perfect description of "toxic garbage." Hopefully your Food Tree is too solid for that solid stuff.

Finally, nuts and peanut butter are mostly oils and should be treated as fat exchanges.

Three things to understand:

1) GI is not a precise number, it indicates a general neighborhood.
2) GI is related to the amounts you eat.
3) GI is influenced by what else you eat.

You want to build your food tree looking at GI patterns.

Look at the Food Tree. It keeps GI comfortably in low range every meal, and keeps your body writing the perfect G-I curve.

The Nutrition and Glycemic Index Guide

Most foodstuffs you need are in this table. They're listed in groups, proteins first. A working knowledge of the GI of what you eat is crucial to keeping your G-I curve healthy. The carbs are therefore annotated with GI information. The first number before each carb is how much in grams of a carb yields 50 grams of sugar, the next number is the GI of that carb. The number after the serving size is the most practical one, because it represents how much that serving will raise your GI. Your goal is to keep your GI well below 40 every meal.

We won't list every concoction of processed products. Whatever their GI, they aren't food groups of the Food Tree because of their content of hidden sugars and harmful fats. They're the additive top tree branches that you eat in the same spirit (pardon the pun) as you drink spirits.

Again, since complete tables are not available, the serving sizes and their GI have been extrapolated from nutritional guides and from actual groceries, and are not precise numbers, but guidelines for developing eating patterns.

GI and Serving sizes: Almost all GI tables give servings in grams. I've made some loose translations to English measurement to give you a feel for how much a serving of the various carbs is. Volume measures are even easier. Think of an 8 oz. cup and divide it up to get the average serving: 4 oz. is generally half a cup, etc. Two oz. of grains is generally ¼ to ⅓ cup. Low density increases the volume, and the density of cereals is so low that 1 oz. fills a cup, GI around 35.

If you look at trends, you'll see that a small serving of sugar or grain-based carb is above 20 for a serving, whereas a piece of fruit will keep your GI around 10. Veggies and dairy work well to keep your GI below 40 for the meal.

Lean Proteins

Lean Meats / Other Lean Proteins:

(7 grams protein, 3 grams fat, and 50 calories per serving) **Serving Size**

Beef	all lean cuts of beef: Roast, round, extra lean ground round, flank steak, fillet mignon	1 oz.
Cottage cheese	non-fat or low-fat	2 oz .
Cheese	non -fat or low-fat	1 oz.
Chicken	skin, fat removed	1 oz.
Egg substitute		2 oz.
Fish	all fresh or frozen	1 oz.
Lamb	chops, shanks, leg	1 oz.
Pork	lean cuts of pork : chops, Canadian bacon, ham, etc.	1 oz.
Ricotta cheese	non-fat or low-fat	2 oz.
Sausage	non-fat or low-fat	1 oz.
Shellfish	clams, crab, lobster, scallops, shrimp	1 oz.
Tofu		2 oz.
Tuna	fresh or canned in water	1 oz .
Turkey	skin removed	1 oz.
Veal	lean chops or roast	1 oz.

Note on serving size: Three ounces meat or fish equals a serving the size of a deck of cards, which equals 20 grams of protein.

Lean Dairy with Carbs:

(12 grams carbohydrate, 8 grams protein, 1 gram fat, and 100 calories per serving)

Grams for GI	GI Value	Skim Milk/Skim-Milk Products	Serving Size	GI of Serving
1000 g	30	Skim (non-fat or low-fat)	8 oz.	7
1000 g	30	Buttermilk (non-fat or low-fat)	8 oz.	7
1000 g	30	Soy milk	8 oz.	7
1000 g	30	Yogurt (non-fat or low-fat, fruited, artificially sweetened)	8 oz.	7

Note on serving size: One ounce of milk or yogurt has 1 gram of protein.

Medium-Fat Proteins

Medium-Fat Meats/Other Medium-Fat Proteins:

(7 grams protein, 5 grams fat, and 75 calories per serving)   **Serving Size**

Beef	most cuts	1 oz.
Cheese	low-fat, part skim	1 oz.
Egg		1 egg
Lamb	most cuts	1 oz.
Liver		1 oz.
Pork	most cuts	1 oz.
Veal	cutlet, ground or cubed, unbreaded	1 oz.

Note on serving size: Three ounces meat or fish equals a serving the size of a deck of cards, which equals 20 grams of protein.

Low-Fat Dairy with Carbs:

(12 grams carbohydrate, 8 grams protein, 3 or more grams of fat, and 120–150 calories per serving)

Grams for GI	GI Value	Skim Milk/Skim-Milk Products	Serving Size	GI of Serving
1000 g	30	Milk (2%)	8 oz.	7
1000 g	30	Yogurt (2%, low-fat, plain)	8 oz.	7

One ounce of milk or yogurt has 1 gram of protein.

High-Fat Proteins

High-Fat Meats/Other High-Fat Proteins:

(7 grams protein, 8 grams fat, and 100 calories per serving)

LIMITED INTAKE		Serving Size
Cheese	regular	1 oz.
Corned beef		1 oz.
Hot dogs		1 oz.
Lunch meats		1 oz.
Prime rib		1 oz.
Sausage		1 oz.
Spareribs		1 oz.

Note on serving size: Three ounces meat or fish equals a serving the size of a deck of cards, which equals 20 grams of protein.

Full-Fat Dairy with Carbs:

(12 grams carbohydrate, 8 grams protein, 5 or more grams of fat, and 150–170 calories per serving)

Grams for GI	GI Value	Skim Milk/Skim-Milk Products	Serving Size	GI of Serving
1000 g	30	Milk (whole)	8 oz.	7
1000 g	30	Yogurt (regular, plain)	8 oz.	7

One ounce of milk or yogurt has 1 gram of protein.

Vegetables/Legumes

Cook vegetables al dente.

Vegetables—Serving Size: 1 cup:

(5 grams carbohydrate, and 25 calories per serving)

GI Value	Vegetable	GI Value	Vegetable
low	Artichoke	low	Jicama
low	Asparagus	low	Mushrooms
low	Bamboo sprouts	low	Okra
low	Bean sprouts	10	Onion
low	Broccoli	low	Peppers (red, green,
low	Brussels sprouts		orange, yellow)
low	Cabbage	low	Radish
low	Cauliflower	low	Sauerkraut
low	Celery	low	Spinach
low	Chicory	low	Summer squash
low	Cucumber	15	Tomatoes
15	Eggplant	low	Turnip
15	All greens (salad, mustard,	low	V8/Tomato juice
	etc.)	low	Water chestnut
10	Green beans	low	Zucchini

Legumes/Starchy/Root Vegetables:

(15 grams carbohydrate, and 80 calories per serving)

GI for GI	GI Value	Legume/Starchy/Root Vegetable	Serving Size	GI of Serving
300 g	30	Beans	3.5 oz.	10
350 g	70	Beans mashed	4.0 oz.	23
150 g	65	Beets	1.5 oz.	21
715 g	30	Carrots, raw	8 oz.	10
830 g	85	Carrots, cooked	9 oz.	28
300 g	55	Corn	3 oz.	17
230 g	22	Peas	2.5 oz.	7
360 g	60	Potato	4 oz.	20
600 g	15	Soy Beans	7 oz.	5
250 g	55	Sweet potato	3 oz.	18
715 g	75	Winter squash	8 oz.	25

Fats

Unsaturated Fats:

(15 grams fat, and 150 calories per serving)

GI Value	Fat	Serving Size
0	Olive oil	1 Tbsp.
0	Vegetable oils (corn, cottonseed, soybean sunflower, safflower, peanut)	1 Tbsp.
0	Avocado	1/2 avocado
0	Mayonnaise (regular)	1 Tbsp.
low	Nuts	10–15
0	Olives	10–15
low	Peanut butter	1 Tbsp.
0	Salad dressing (regular)	2 Tbsp.
0	Seeds	1 Tbsp.

Saturated Fats:

(15 grams fat, and 100 calories per serving)

GI Value	Fat	Serving Size
0	Bacon	3 slices
0	Butter	1 Tbsp.
0	Cream (whipping)	2.5 Tbsp.
0	Cream cheese	3 Tbsp.
0	Sour cream	6 Tbsp.

High-Fat Carbohydrate Mixtures

(15 grams carbs, 10 grams fat, and 150 calories per serving)

Grams for GI	GI Value	Fat	Serving Size	GI of Serving
80 g	65	Candy bar	1 oz.	21
150 g	22	Dark chocolate	1.5 oz.	7
150 g	75	French fries	1.5 oz.	25
200 g	60	Ice cream	2 oz.	20
100g	55	Potato chips	1 oz.	18
100 g	50	Scones, muffins, biscuits	1 oz.	17

Fruits

Fresh Fruits:
(15 grams carbohydrate, and 60 calories per serving)

Grams for GI	GI Value	Fruit	Serving Size	GI of Serving
420 g	40	Apple	5 oz.	13
500 g	57	Apricot	6 oz.	19
250 g	60	Banana	3 oz.	20
2 lbs.	20	Blackberries, blueberries, raspberries	10 oz.	6
2 lbs.	65	Cantaloupe, honeydew melon	10 oz.	21
500 g	22	Cherries	6 oz.	7
350 g	25	Grapefruit	4 oz .	8
313 g	45	Grapes	3.5 oz.	15
500g	53	Kiwi	6 oz.	17
350 g	50	Mango	4 oz.	16
550 g	44	Orange	6.5 oz.	14
350 g	60	Papaya	4 oz.	20
500g	40	Peach, nectarine	6 oz.	13
500g	35	Pear	6 oz.	11
240 g	60	Pineapple	3 oz.	20
500g	40	Plum	6 oz.	13
2 lbs.	40	Strawberries	10 oz.	13
2 lbs.	72	Watermelon	10 oz.	25

Dried Fruits:

Grams for GI	GI Value	Fruit	Serving Size	GI of Serving
100g	31	Apricots	1 oz.	10
90 g	30	Prunes (medium)	1 oz.	15
70 g	75	Raisins	0.67 oz.	25

Fruits (continued)

Fruit Juices/Sugary Drinks:

Grams for GI	GI Value	Fruit Juice/Sugary Drink	Serving Size	GI of Serving
450 g	40	Apple juice	5.5 oz.	10
500 g	40	Carrot juice	6 oz.	10
450 g	40	Grapefruit juice	5.5 oz.	10
450 g	50	Orange juice	5.5 oz.	10
1200 g	38	Tomato juice	13 oz.	12
450 g	60	Cola drinks	5.5 oz.	20
450 g	78	Gatorade®	5.5 oz.	26

Refined Carbohydrates

Sugars:

(15 grams carbohydrate, and 60 calories per serving)

Gr ams for GI	GI Value	Sugar	Serving Size	GI of Serving
50 g	100	Glucose	1 Tbsp.	33
50 g	70	Sucrose (table sugar)	1 Tbsp.	23
50 g	23	Fructose	1 Tbsp.	8
63 g	60	Honey	1 Tbsp.	20
70 g	50	Jam	1 Tbsp.	17
1000 g	105	Beer	10 oz.	35
60 g	70	Corn syrup	1 Tbsp.	23
60 g	70	Maple syrup	1 Tbsp.	23

Starches:

Note: The protein in grain is incomplete.

(15 grams carbohydrate, 3 grams protein, 1 gram fat, and 80 calories per serving)

Gr ams for GI	GI Value	Starch	Serving Size	GI of Serving
86 g	85	White flour	1 oz.	28
94 g	70	Whole wheat	1 oz.	23
70 g	70	Polenta	0.75 oz.	23
80 g	60	Oatmeal	0.75 oz.	30
80 g	30	Oat bran	0.75 oz.	10
60 g	70	Shredded wheat	0.67 oz.	23
60 g	85	Dry cereal	0.67 oz.	28
180 g	22	Whole barley	2 oz.	7
105 g	50	Cracked barley	1.5 oz.	15
280 g	35	Quinoa	3 oz.	12
220 g	40	Macaroni, noodles, spaghetti and other pasta, cooked	2.5 oz.	13
300 g	50	Bulgur	3.5 oz.	16
220 g	55	Corn	2.5 oz.	18
260 g	45	Pasta (white)	3 oz.	15
290 g	40	Pasta (dark)	3.5 oz.	13

Refined Carbohydrates (continued)

Starches

Note: The protein in grain is incomplete.

(15 grams carbohydrate, 3 grams protein, 1 gram fat, and 80 calories per serving)

Gr ams for GI	GI Value	Starch	Serving Size	GI of Serving
350 g	60	Potato (whole, boiled)	4 oz.	20
250 g	85	Potato (peeled, boiled)	3 oz.	28
200 g	85	Potato (baked)	2.5 oz.	28
350 g	90	Potato (mashed, instant)	4 oz.	30
220 g	45	Rice (white)	2.5 oz.	15
220 g	55	Rice (brown)	2.5 oz.	17
220 g	35	Rice (wild)	2.5 oz.	11
330 g	35	Mung beans	4 oz.	8

Breads:

Note: The protein in grain is incomplete.

(15 grams carbohydrate, 3 grams protein, 1 gram fat, and 80 calories per serving)

Grams for GI	GI Value	Starch	Serving Size	GI of Serving
110 g	70	Breads (whole-wheat, rye, white, raisin, other)	1 slice=1 oz.	23
110 g	50	Pumpernickel	1 slice=1 oz.	16
100 g	70	Bagel, bun, roll, or tortilla	½ bagel, bun	23
125 g	48	Oatmeal bread	1 slice=1 oz.	16
70 g	75	Graham crackers	0.75 oz.	25
85 g	80	Pretzels	0.75 oz.	27
100 g	55	Popcorn	1 oz.	18
200 g	60	Pizza	2 oz.	20

Free Foods

Condiments:
Dill pickles (unsweetened)
Horseradish
Hot sauce
Vinegar

Drinks:
Bouillon/broth (non-fat)
Cocoa powder (unsweetened, baking
   type) [1 Tbsp.]
Coffee/tea
Soft drinks (calorie-free including
   carbonated drinks)

Seasonings:
Flavoring extracts (vanilla, almond,
   butter, etc.)
Garlic/garlic powder
(All) Herbs (fresh or dried)
Lemon/lemon juice
(All) Spices
Soy sauce
Worcestershire sauce

Sweet Substitutes:
Gelatin (sugar-free)
Jam/jelly (sugar-free) [2 tsp.]

Sources of Vitamins

Vitamin	Source
Vitamin A	Highly pigmented (yellow, orange, red, dark green) vegetables, dairy
Vitamin B	Meats, organ meats, dairy, eggs, legumes, green vegetables , whole grains
Vitamin C	All fruits, especially citrus
Vitamin D	Sunlight on the skin, salmon, dairy
Vitamin E	Vegetable seed oil, wheat-germ oil
Vitamin K	Broccoli, cabbage, lettuce; formed by bacteria in your colon
Folate	Leafy vegetables, beans
Trace minerals	Fruits and vegetables
Flavonoids	Fruits and vegetables
Fiber	Fruits and vegetables, whole grains, legumes

Calorie Expenditure Chart

Activity	Calories expended per hour
Lying, sitting, computer work, studying, office work	less than 100
Light: house work, puttering around the house	100
Walking, golf, spring cleaning, gardening	200
Dancing, swimming, skating, bicycling	300
Moderate: power walking, jogging, aerobics, circuit training, tennis, ball games	400
Hard: aerobics, jumping rope, running, cycling, ball games	500–700

Treats—a list to start you thinking about treats in new ways

1) Yogurt, as long as a serving is less than 130 calories (no added sugar). Add fresh fruit or berries. Low/nonfat cottage cheese or ricotta works well too.

2) Keep low-fat cheese sticks or beef jerky on hand for quick snacks. (Easy on dried salted meats if you have blood-pressure issues.)

3) Use sugar-free Jell-O. Top it with a little whipped cream for an extra treat. Mix them and you have a mousse. Sugar-free chocolate pudding is available as well.

4) A cafe latte/cappuccino with non/low-fat milk.

5) Tomato and mozzarella slices make a wonderful Caprese salad.

6) Make veggie or meat omelets with egg whites/egg substitutes.

7) Make a great coleslaw, add apples for interest, and just limit the dressing.

8) Make a tasty dip with equal parts of nonfat sour cream and nonfat yogurt; add your favorite dip flavor. Or try equal parts of nonfat cottage cheese and your favorite salsa. Eat on "chips" of bell pepper, cucumber, or celery.

9) Treat yourself to a portion of gulf shrimp with cocktail sauce, or some scallops or oysters if those tempt you.

10) Wrap your sandwich meat in lettuce instead of bread.

11) Put celery/carrot sticks in a small glass with ranch or other dressing at the bottom. Very antipasto.

12) Olives and nuts make wonderful nibbles. Small quantities go a long way, though, since they exchange against your olive oil (see nutrition guide). Very Mediterranean.

13) Eat your cheese and crackers plus fruit and minus the crackers (pick a lower-fat cheese). Very Continental.

14) A high-quality protein bar will give you 15 grams of protein while being decadent enough to stop you eating candy.

Now We'll Make You an Intuitive Chef

Do what great chefs do: buy what's in season, and think about how you're going to prepare it later.

I cook by "a dash of this and a little of that." If that doesn't work for you, consult a basic cookbook in the beginning.

Have good olive oil and butter on hand. Use them sparingly. Flavored vinegars and herbs give interesting variations to dishes. Sprinkle grated Parmesan or other cheese on dishes. They add flavor and fullness. Sprinkle nuts on desserts for texture and flavor. Snack on hard cheeses, olives, and crudités.

Fish and meat freeze well for a short time. Buy your dinners for the week and freeze them. Pull one out every morning and it will be ready to cook when you come home.

Breakfast

Make it simple: eggs, lean breakfast meats, Canadian bacon, ham, low-fat cheese, yogurt, cottage cheese, protein bars, fruits, berries, tomatoes, onion, mushrooms, tomato/V8 juice.

Sunday brunch

Dr. Elvebakk's anytime frittata: dice any two or three vegetables, lunch meats, and dinner leftovers; sauté with olive oil in a nonstick pan.

Crack and mix two to three egg whites per person, only one yolk if you're watching your cholesterol, a dash of milk, salt, and pepper. Add a dash of hot pepper or other spice/herb if you like. Pour over vegetable/meat mix. Reduce heat, cover, and cook till done.

Mrs. B's Easy Pancakes

½ cup cottage cheese

1 egg

2 tablespoons flour

Mix and cook in medium nonstick pan with a little olive oil or butter. Eat with butter and a little reduced-sugar jam or syrup. This yummy breakfast packs some 20 grams of protein and minimal carbs.

Lunch

Put lunchmeats, chicken, turkey, shellfish, cheese, cottage cheese, and tofu on a bed of lettuce, spinach, grated cabbage, carrots, avocado, tomato, and cucumber. Or wrap in lettuce as a sandwich.

A creative result can come out of almost any combination of what's in your refrigerator.

Dinner

Make it easy. Get a roasted chicken, add seasonings, eat what you need, and freeze the rest. Steam up a pot of veggies (mix a couple of colors). Total 10–15 minutes, and a delicious, nutritious dinner instead of a disaster meal of fat and sugar. Like your veggies stir-fried? Buy a cheese plane, slice your veggies thin, and stir-fry them in a tablespoon of olive oil. Add salt, pepper, and rice-wine or other vinegar. Bravo!

Buy a grill pan. Use it for fish and meat. It takes minutes and gives you restaurant results. Grill low-fat sausages along with peppers and onions brushed with olive oil for a wonderful one-pan meal.

Grill any meat/fish/vegetable and add flavors: salsa, herbs, spices, sauces. Applause, please.

For starch use legumes such as peas, beans, and squash. They add lots of fiber and flavor. Liven them up with oil-vinegar combinations, garlic, mustard, lemon juice, herbs, and spices.

The Grand Gourmet: Sauté chicken breasts or pork medallions in olive oil, garlic, and salt/pepper. Add white wine or lemon juice to pan. Add your favorite fruit or berries. Cover and cook till chicken is done. Open a bag of mixed greens. Dress with olive oil and your favorite vinegar. Delicious.

The same money and minimal effort, but you're living so much better. Once you get used to eating good food, you and your family will reject the low quality of fast food.

Dessert

Cut up your favorite fruits and add yogurt flavored with a little fruit juice, lemon or lime juice, mint, cinnamon, or other flavor.

Gourmet: Sauté your favorite fruit or berries with butter in a pan. Add orange or other liqueur. Reduce slightly and serve. Add a dollop of yogurt if you like. Yummy and easy.

My Mother's Bread

Very chewy, delicious, and GI about 15 for one slice. Lots of soluble oat fiber.

4 cups rolled oats

1 cup white flour

2 cups coarse milled whole-wheat flour

4 tablespoons olive oil or butter

2 packages dry yeast

2 cups water

Put it all in your bread maker.

By hand: Warm water oil/butter and yeast to about 90° F. (lukewarm). Dissolve yeast.

Mix all flour, add liquid, and work into a soft dough. Let rest in a warm place for 2 hours. Rework dough into two loaves. Put into loaf pan. Let rest for 30 minutes in warm place. Bake for 35 minutes in a preheated oven at 400°F.

Hankering for a cool drink? Here's *Teri's Happy-Hour Margarita*.

¼ tub crystal light lemonade (sugar- and GI-free)

1 cup water

1 cup tequila

Juice of two limes

Ice

Mix/blend

EPILOGUE

I close remembering my Viking ancestor King "Holy" Olav and his standard-bearer Tord Foleson fighting to introduce Christianity to those heathen Scandinavians in the battle of Stiklestad in 1030. They lost the battle, but obviously won the war. In loose translation from the poem by Per Sivle:

Men may fall
But the standard must
As witness into the ground be thrust.
And that is the glory of it all
The standard stands though the man may fall.

BIBLIOGRAPHY

Agus, M. S. D., J. E. Swain, C. L. Larson, et al. Dietary composition and physiological adaptations to energy restriction. *Am J Clin Nutr, 71,* (2000), 901–07.

Alberti, K. G., P. Zimmet, J. Shaw. The Metabolic Syndrome–a new worldwide definition. *Lancet, 366, (2005), 1059.*

Allison, D. B. et al. Annual deaths attributable to obesity in the United States. JAMA, 282, (1999), 1530–38.

American College of Sports Medicine. American College of Sports Medicine Position Stand. The recommended quantity and quality of exercise for developing and maintaining cardiorespiratory and muscular fitness, and flexibility, in healthy adults. Med Sci Sports Exerc, 30, (1998), 975–91.

Andreasen. Brave New Brain: Conquering Mental Illness in the Era of the Genome. Oxford University Press, 2001.

Appel, L. J., F. M. Sacks, V. J. Carey, et al. Effects of Protein, Monosaturated Fat and Carbohydrate Intake on Blood Pressure and Serum Lipids. JAMA, 294, (2005), 455–64.

Atkins, Robert Dr. Dr. Atkins' Diet Revolution. Bantam Books, 1972.

Atkinson, William Walker. Thought Vibration, or the Law of Attraction in the Thought World. Digireads.com Publishing

Benson H. The Maximum Mind. Random House, 1987.

Berrigan D., K. Dodd, R. P. Trolano, et al. Patterns of health behavior in US adults. Prev Med, 36, (2003), 615–23.

Blackburn, G. L., W. A. Walker. Science-based solutions to obesity: what are the roles of academia, government, industry and health care? Am J Clin Nutr, 82, (2005), 207S–10S.

Blair, S. N., T. S. Church. The fitness, obesity and health equation: is physical activity the common denominator? JAMA, 292, (2004), 1232–34.

Boyle, J. P., A. A. Honeycutt, K. M. Narayan, et al. Projection of diabetes through 2050: impact on changing demography and disease prevalence in the US. Diabetes Care, 24, (2001), 1936–40.

Bray, G. A. Medical Consequences of Obesity. Journal of Clinical Endocrinology, 89 (6), (2004), 2583–89.

Brown, A. A., HU FB. Dietary modulation of endothelial function. Implications for cardiovascular disease. Am J Clin Nutr, 73, (2001), 673–86.

Burke, V., J. M. Hodgson, L. J. Bellin, et al. Dietary protein and soluble fiber reduce ambulatory blood pressure in treated hypertensives. Hypertension, 38, (2001), 821–26.

Carbohydrate Intake on Blood Pressure and Serum Lipids. JAMA, 294, (2005), 2455–64.

Cardenas, G. A., C. J. Lavie. How Significant is Low HDL Cholesterol? Emergency Medicine, September 2005.

Carroll, M. D., D. A. Lacher, P. D. Sorlie, et al. Trends in Serum Lipids and Lipoproteins of Adults, 1960–2002l. JAMA, 294, (2005), 1773–81.

Centers for Disease Control and Prevention. Prevalence of physical activity including lifestyle activities among adults. Morbidity and Mortality Weekly Report. 52, (2003), 764–69.

Chanmugam, P. et al. Did fat intake in the United States really decline between 1989–1991? and Boyle, J. P., A. A. Honeycutt, K. M. Narayan, et al. Projection of diabetes burden through 2050: Impact of changing demography and disease prevalence in the US. Diabetes Care, 24, (2001), 1936–40.

Chobanian, A. V., G. L. Bakris, H. R. Black et al. The Seventh Report of the Joint National Committee on Prevention, Detection, Evaluation and Treatment of High Blood Pressure: the JNC 7 report. JAMA, 289, (2003), 2560.

Christakis, N. A., J. H. Fowler. The Spread of Obesity in Large Social Network. NEJM, 357, (2007), 370–79.

Christakis, D. A. The Hidden and Potent Effects of Television Advertising. JAMA, 295, (2006), 1.

Clark, M. M., V. Pera, M. G. Goldstein, et al. Counseling strategies for obese patients. Am J Preventive Med, 12, (1996), 266–70.

Cutler, J. A., E. Obarzanek. Nutrition and blood pressure: is protein one link toward a strategy of hypertension prevention. Ann Intern Med, 143, (2005), 74–75.

Davis, P. G., S. D. Phinney. Differential effect of two very low calorie diets on aerobic and anaerobic performance. Int J of Obesity, 14, (1990), 779–87.

Deschenes, M. R., W. J. Kraemer. Performance and physiological adaptations to resistance training. Am J Phys Med Rehab, 81, (2002), S3–S16.

Drohan, S. H. Managing early childhood obesity in the primary care setting: a behavior modification approach. Ped Nursing, 28, (2002), 599–610.

Eaton, S. B., M. Shostak, M. Konner. The Paleolithic Prescription. New York: Harper and Row, 1988.

Eaton, S. B., S. B. Eaton III, M. J. Konner. Paleolithic nutrition revisited, a twelve-year retrospective on its nature and implications. Eur J Clin Nutr, 51, (1997), 207–16.

Ehrman, D. A., R. B. Barnes, R. L. Rosenfield, et al. Prevalence of impaired glucose tolerance and diabetes in women with polycystic ovary syndrome. Diabetes Care, 22, (1999), 141–45.

Feigenbaum, M. S., M. L. Pollock. Strength training rationale for current guidelines for adult fitness programs. Physical Sportsmed, 25, (1997), 44–64.

Ferrara, L. A., A. S. Raimond, et al. Olive oil and reduced need for antihypertensive medications. Arch Intern Med, 80, (2000), 837–42.

Festa, A., Tracy P. D'Agostino Jr., et al. C-reactive protein is more strongly related to post-glucose load than to fasting glucose in non-diabetic subjects: the Insulin Resistance Atherosclerotic Study. Diabetes Med, 19, (2002), 939–43.

Finn, S. Now and again: the food and beverage industry demonstrates its commitment to a healthy America. Am J Clin Nutr, 82, (2005), 253S–55S.

Fletcher, G. F., G. K. Balady, E. A. Amsterdam, et al. Exercise standards for testing and training: a statement for health care professionals from the American Heart Association. Circulation 2001, 104, 1694–1740.

Fontaine, K. R., D. T. Redden, C. Wang, et al: Years of life lost due to obesity. JAMA, 289, (2003), 187–93.

Forbes.com, 2/27/06. IMS Health: America's Top Selling Drugs–a Who's Who of blockbusters.

Ford, E. S., M. A. Ford, J. C. Will, et al. Achieving a healthy lifestyle among United States adults: a long way to go. Ethn Dis, 11, (2001), 224–31.

Foster, G. A., A. P. Makris, B. A. Bailer. Behavioral treatment of obesity. AM J Clin Nutr, 82, (2005), 230S–35S.

Foster, G. D., H. R. Wyatt, J. O. Hill, et al. A randomized trial of a low carbohydrate diet for obesity. N Engl J Med, 348, (2003), 2082–90.

Foster-Powell, K., S. H. Holt, J. C. Brand-Miller. International table of glycemic index and glycemic load values. Am J Clin Nutr, 76, (2002), 5–56.

Gerstenblith, G. *Cardiovascular Aging: What We Can Learn From Caloric Restriction.* J Am Coll Cardiol, 47, (2006), 403–04.

Ginsberg, H. N. *Non pharmacological management of low levels of high density lipoprotein cholesterol.* Am J Cardiol, 86, (2000), L41–45.

Ginsberg, H. N. *Treatment for patients with the metabolic syndrome.* Am J Cardiol, 91, (2003), 29E–39E.

Glascow, R. E., E. G. Eakin, S. J. Bacac, et al. *Physician advice and support for physical activity: Results from a national survey.* Am J Prev Med, 21, (2001), 189–96.

Goldberg, R. J., M. Larson, D. Levy. *Factors Associated with Survival to 75 Years of Age in Middle-aged Men and Women.* Arch Intern Med, 156, (1996), 505–09.

Grodstein, F., R. Levine, L. Troy, et al. *Three-Year Follow up of Participants in a commercial Weight Loss Program.* Arch Int Med, 156, (1996), 1302–06.

Grundy, S. M., H. B. Brewer, J. L. Cleeman, et al. *Definition of metabolic syndrome. Report of the National Heart, Lung and Blood Institute/American Heart Association conference on scientific issues relating to definition.* 109, (2004), 433–38.

Grundy, S. M., J. I. Cleeman, S. R. Daniels, et al. *Diagnosis and management of the metabolic syndrome. An American Heat Association/National Heart, Lung and Blood Institute Scientific Statement,* 112, (2005), 2735.

Halton, T. L., F. B. Hu. *The effects of high protein diets on thermogenesis, satiety and weight loss: a critical review.* J Coll Nutr, 23(5), (2004), 373–85.

Hatzianfreu, E. I., J. P. Koplan, M. C. Weinstein, et al. *A cost-effectiveness analysis of exercise as a health promotion activity.* Am J Public Health, 78, (1988), 1417–21.

Health affairs. *The Policy Journal of the Health Sphere. Data Watch: The Effects of Obesity, Smoking and Drinking On Medical Problems and Costs.* Vol. 21, no 2.

Healthy People 2010. US Department of Health and Human Services, 2003.

Isomaa, B. *A major health hazard: the metabolic syndrome.* Life Sci, 73 (19), (2003), 2395–411.

Jackicic, J. M., A. D. Otto. *Physical activity considerations for the treatment and prevention of obesity.* Am J Clin Nutr, 82, 2005, 2265S–69S.

Jarvi, A. E., B. E. Karlstrom, Y. E. Granfeldt, et al. *Improved Glycemic Control and lipid Profile and Normalized Fibrinolytic Activity on a Low Glycemic Index Diet in Type 2 Diabetic patients.* Diabetes Care, 22, (1999), 10–18.

Jeffery, R. W., R. R. Wing, Thorson, et al. Strengthening behavioral interventions for weight loss: a randomized trial of food provision and monetary incentives. J Consult Clin Psychol, 6, (1993), 1038–45.

Keesey, R. E., and M. D. Hirvonen. Body Weight Set Points and Adjustment. Journ of Nutr, 127, (1997), 1875–83S.

Khaw, K. T., N. Wareham, R. Luben, et al. Glycated hemoglobin, diabetes and mortality in men in Norfolk cohort of European prospective investigation of cancer and nutrition. British Med Journal, 322, (2001), 15–18.

Korner, J., R. L. Leibel. To Eat or Not to Eat—How the Gut Talks to the Brain. New Engl. J Med, 349, (2003), 926–28.

Krauss, R. M., P. J. Blanche, R. S. Rawlings, et al. Separate effects of reduced carbohydrate intake and weight loss on atherogenic dyslipidemia. *Am J Clin Nutr, 83, (2006), 1025–31.*

Kris-Etherton, P. M., W. S. Harris, J. L. Appel, et al. Fish consumption, fish oil, omega-3 fatty acids, and cardiovascular disease. Circulation 2002, 106, 2747–57.

Last, A. R., S. A. Wilson. Low Carbohydrate Diets. American Family Physician (2006), 73, 1942–48.

Layman, D. K., J. I. Baum. Dietary protein impact on glycemic control during weight loss. J Nutr, 134 (4), (2004), 968S–73S.

Layman, D. K., R. A. Boileau, D. J. Erickson, et al. A reduced ratio of carbohydrate to protein improves body composition and blood lipid profiles during weight loss in adults. J Nutr, 133, (2003), 411–17.

Layman, D. K, H. Shiue, C. Sather, et al. Increased dietary protein modifies glucose and insulin homeostasis in adult women during weight loss. J Nutr, 133, (2003), 405–10.

Layman, D. K. The role of leucine in weight loss diets and glucose homeostasis. J Nutr, 133, (2003) 261S–67S.

Lee, I. M., R. S. Paffenberger Jr., C. H. Hennekens, et al. Physical activity, physical fitness and longevity. Aging (Milano), 9, (1997), 2–11.

Lemon, W. R. Is increased Dietary Protein Necessary or Beneficial for Individuals with Physically Active Lifestyle? Nutr Rev, (II) S, (1996), 169–S75.

Lew, Garfinkel. Obesity and Mortality Risk. J Chron Disease, 32, (1979), 563–76.

Lieb, C. W. The Effects on Human Beings of a Twelve Months' Exclusive Meat Diet. JAMA, July 6, 1929.

Liu, S., et al. Relationship between a diet with high glycemic load and plasma concentration of high sensitivity C-reactive protein in middle-aged women. Am J Clin Nutr, 75, (2002), 492–98.

Liu, S., M. J. Willett, F. B. Stampfer, et al. A prospective study of dietary glycemic load and risk of myocardial infarction in women. Am J Clin Nutr, 75, (2002), 492–98.

Ludwig, D. S. Dietary Glycemic Index and Obesity. J Nut, 130, (2000), 280S–83S.

Manson, J. E., P. J. Skerrett, P. Greenland, et al. The escalating pandemic of obesity and sedentary life style. A call to action for clinicians. Arch Int Med, 164, (2004), 249–58.

Marchesini, G., M. Brizi, A. M. Morselli Labate, et al. Association of non alcoholic liver fatty disease with insulin resistance. Am J Med, 107 (5), (1999), 450–55.

Marcus, B. H., J. S. Rossi, V. C. Selby, et al. The stages and processes of exercise adoption and maintenance in a worksite example. Health Psychology, 11, (1992), 386–95.

McGuire, M. T., R. R. Wing, M. L. Klem, et al. Behavioral strategies of individuals who have maintained long term weight losses. Obes Research, 7, (1999), 334–41.

McGuire, M. T., R. R. Wing, M. L. Klem, et al. What predicts weight regain among a group of successful weight losers? J Consult Clin Psychol, 67, (1999), 177–85.

Mohanty, P. J., W. Hamouda, R. Garg, et al. Glucose challenge stimulates reactive oxygen species (ROS) generated by leucocytes. J Clin Metabolism, 85, (2000), 2970–73.

Mora, S, M. B. S. S. Min Lee, J. E. Buring, et al. Association of Physical Activity and Body Mass Index With Novel and Traditional Cardiovascular Biomarkers in Women. JAMA, 295, (2006), 1412–19.

Morris, M. C., D. A. Evans, J. L. Bienias, et al. Consumption of fish and n-3 fatty acids and risk of incident Alzheimer disease. Arch Neurol, 60, (2003), 940–46.

Naldi, L., F. Parazzini, L. Peli, et al. Dietary factors and the risk of psoriasis. Results of an Italian case-controlled study. British Journal of Dermatology, 134, (1996), 101–06.

Narbro, K. et al. Pharmaceutical costs in obese individuals: a comparison with a randomly selected population sample and long-term changes after conventional and surgical treatment: the SOS intervention study. Arch Intern Med, 162, (2002), 2061–69.

Neuschwander-Tetri, B. A., S. H. Caldwell. Non–alcoholic steatohepatitis: summary of an AASLD Single Topic Conference. Hepatology, 37 (5), (2003), 1202–19.

Noakes, M., P. R. Foster, J. B. Keogh, et al. Meal replacements are as effective as structured weight-loss diets for treating obesity in adults with features of metabolic syndrome. J Nutr, 134, (2004;), 1894–99.

Obesity tops smoking as a risk. Report of the RAND Institute, Santa Monica, Calif. Los Angeles Associated Press, June 2000.

O'Keefe, J. H. Jr., L. Cordain. Cardiovascular disease resulting from a diet at odds with our Paleolithic genome: How to become a 21st Century Hunter-Gatherer. Review. Mayo Clin Proc, 79, (2004), 101–03.

Ogden, C. L. Carroll, M.D., L. R. Curtin, et al. Prevalence of Overweight and Obesity in the United States 1999–2004. JAMA, 295, (20063), 1549–76.

Park, S. K., et al. The effect of combined aerobic and resistance exercise training on abdominal fat in obese middle-aged women. J Physiol Anthropol Appl Human Sci, 22, (2003), 129–35.

Pate, R. R., M. Pratt, S. N. Blair, et al. Physical activity and public health. A recommendation from the Centers for Disease Control; and Prevention and the American College of Sports Medicine. JAMA, 273, (1995), 402–07.

Penbrey, M., L. O. Bygren, G.P. Kaati, et al. Sex-specific sperm-mediated transgenerational responses in humans. Hum Genet, 14, (2005), 159–166.

Phelan, S., J. O. Hill, W. Lang, et al. Recovery from relapse among successful weight maintainers. Am J Clin Nutr, 78, (2003), 1079–84.

Philipson, T. Government perspective: food labeling. Am J Clin Nutr, 82, (2005), 262S–64S.

Pollock, M. I., B. A. Franklin, G. J. Balady, et al. AHA Science Advisory: Resistance exercise in individuals with or without cardiovascular disease: benefits, rationale, safety, and prescription. An advisory from the Committee on Exercise, Rehabilitation, and Prevention. Council on Clinical Cardiology, American Heart Association; Position paper endorsed by the American College of Sports Medicine. Circulation 2000, 101, 828–33.

Pories, W. J., M. S. Swanson, K. G. MacDonald, et al. Who would have thought it? An operation proves to be the most effective therapy for adult onset diabetes mellitus. Ann Surg, 222, (1995), 339–50.

Prochaska, J. O., C. C. DiClemente, J. C. Norcross. In search of how people change. American Psychologist, 47, (1992), 1102–13.

Ratuziu, V., et al. Liver fibrosis in overweight patients. Gastroenterology, 118 (6), (2000), 1117.

Reaven, G. M. Banting lecture 1988. Role of insulin resistance in human disease. Diabetes, 37, (1988), 1595–60.

Reeves, J. R., A. P. Rafferty. Healthy Lifestyle Characteristics Among Adults in the United States. 2000. Arch Intern Med, 165, (2000), 854–57.

Rizkalla, S. W., L. Tagbrid, M. Laromiguiere, et al. Improved plasma glucose control, whole body glucose utilization and lipid profile in a low glycemic index diet in type 2 diabetic men: a randomized controlled trial. Diabetes Care, 27, (2004), 1866–72.

Roberts, R. E. et al. Prospective Association between obesity and depression: evidence from the Alameda County Study. Int. Journal of Obesity Related Metabolic Disorders, 27, (2003), 514–21.

Rush, S. R. Exercise prescription for the treatment of medical conditions. Curr Sports Rep, 2, (2003), 159–65.

Samaha, F. F., I. Nayar, P. Seshadri, et al. A low carbohydrate as compared with a low fat diet in severe obesity. N Engl J Med, 348, (2003), 2074–81.

Selvin, E., J. Coresh, S. H. Golden et al. Glycemic Control and Coronary Heart Disease in Persons With and Without Diabetes: The Atherosclerosis Risk in Communities Study. Arch Int Med, 165, (2005), 1910–16.

Short, D. When science meets the consumer: the role of industry Am J Clin Nutr, 82, (2005), 256S–58S.

Sinha, R., et al. Prevalence of impaired glucose tolerance among children and adolescents with marked obesity. New England Journal of Medicine (2002), 346 (11): 802–10.

Spiegel, A. M., B. A. Alving. Executive summary of the Strategic Plan for National Institutes of Health Obesity Research. Am J Clin Nutr, 82, (2002), 2111S–4S.

Stefanick, M. L., S. Mackey, M. Sheehan, et al. Effects of diet and exercise in men and postmenopausal women with low levels of HDL cholesterol and high levels of LDL cholesterol. N Engl J Med, 339, (1998), 12–20.

Steinberger, J., et al. Adiposity in childhood predicts obesity and insulin resistance in young adulthood. J. Pediatr, 138 (4), (2001), 469–73.

St-Onge, M. P., K. L. Keller, and S. B. Heymsfield. Changes in childhood food consumption patterns: a cause for concern in light of increasing body weights. American Journal of Clinical Nutrition, 78 (6), (2003), 1068–73.

Stunkard, A. J., J. Sobal. Psychosocial consequences of obesity. In Eating disorders and obesity: a comprehensive handbook. Ed. K. D. Brownell and C. G. Fairburn. New York: Guilford Press, 1995, 417–21.

Sturm, R. Increases in clinically severe obesity in the United States 1986–2000. Arch Intern Med, 163 (18), (2003), 2146–48.

Szapary, P. O., L. T. Bloedon, G. D. Foster. Physical activity and its effect on lipids. Curr Cardiol Reports, 5, (2003), 488–92.

Terpstra, A. H. M. Effects of conjugated linoleic acid on body composition and plasma lipids in humans: an overview of the literature. Review. Am J Clin Nutr, 47, (2004), 352–61.

Third Report on the National Cholesterol Education Program (NCEP). Expert Panel on Detection, Evaluation and Treatment of High Blood Cholesterol in Adults final report. Circulation 2002, 106, 3143–3421.

Toborek, M., Yong Woo Lee, Rosario Garrido, et al. Unsaturated fatty acids selectively induce an inflammatory environment in human endothelial cells. Am J Clin Nutr, 75, (2002), 119–25.

Tonkin, A. High density lipoprotein cholesterol and treatments guidelines. Am J Cardiol, 88, (2000), 41N–44N.

Tumilehto, J., J. Lindstrom, J. G. Eriksson, et al. Prevention of Type 2 Diabetes Mellitus by Changes in Lifestyle among Subjects with Impaired Glucose Tolerance. N Engl J Med, 334, (2001), 1343–50.

Van Baak, M. A., et al. Leisure-time activity is an important determinant of long term weight maintenance after weight loss in the Sibutramine Trial on Obesity Reduction and Maintenance (STORM trial). Am J Clin Nutr, 78, (2003), 209–14.

Verduin, P., S. Agarwal, S. Waltman. Solutions to obesity: perspectives from the food industry. Am J Clin Nutr, 82, (2005), 259S–61S.

Vernon, M., B. Kueser, M. Transue, et al. Clinical Experience of a Carbohydrate-Restricted Diet for the Metabolic Syndrome. The Bariatrician, fall 2005.

Wadden, T. A., G. D. Foster. Behavioral treatment of obesity. Med Clin Nutr Am, 8, (2000), 441–61.

Wadden, T. A., G. D. Foster. Behavioral treatment of obesity. Med Clin Nutr Am, 84, (2002), 441–62.

Walford, R. L., L. J. Walford. The Anti-Aging Plan. New York: Marlowe & Co., reissued 2005.

Wang, W. E., D. R. Ramey, D. Jared, et al. Postponed Development of Disability in Elderly Runners. Arch Int Med, 162, (2002), 285–94.

Warensjo, E., J. Sundstrom, L. Lind, et al. Factor analysis of fatty acids in serum lipid as a measure of dietary fat quality in relation to the metabolic syndrome in men. Am J Clin Nutr, 84, (2006), 442–48.

Weintraub, M. Long term weight control: Conclusions. Clinical Pharmacology and Therapeutics, 51 (5), (1992), 642–46.

Weiss, R., J. Dziura, T. S. Burger, et al. Obesity and the metabolic syndrome in children and adolescents. New England Journal of Medicine, 350, (2004), 62.

Willett, W., M. Stampfer. Rebuilding the Food Pyramid. Scientific American, January 2003.

Wing, R. R., A. A. Gorin. Behavioral techniques for treating the obese patient. Primary Care, 30, (2003), 375–91.

Wing, R. R., J. O. Hill. Successful weight loss maintenance. Annu Rev Nutr, 21, (2001), 323–41.

Wolfe, B. M., P. M. Giovannetti. High protein diet complements resin therapy of familial hypercholesterolemia. Clin Invest Med, 15, (1992), 349–59.

Wolfe. B. M., L. A. Piche. Replacement of carbohydrate by protein in a conventional-fat diet reduces cholesterol and triglyceride concentrations in healthy normolipic subjects. Clin Invest Med, 22, (1999), 140–48.

Wu, T., E. Giovanni, T. Pischon, et al. Fructose, glycemic load and quantity and quality of carbohydrate in relation to plasma C-peptide in US women. Am J Clin Nutr, 80, (2004), 1043–49.

Zhang, H. Y., S. Reddy, T. A. Kotchen. A high sucrose, high linoleic acid diet potentiates hypertension in Dahl salt sensitive rat. Am J Hypertens, 12, (1999) 183–87.

Made in the USA